Don't Necessarily Trust Me, I'm a Doctor

Don't Necessarily Trust Me, I'm a Doctor

From a married couple of family practitioners with over 45 years of practice in the same community:

A ROAD MAP TO FINDING A TRUSTWORTHY HEALTHCARE PROVIDER AND AVOIDING THE DANGERS OF NOT DOING SO

JUDSON HENDERSON, M.D
PATRICIA HENDERSON, FNP-BC

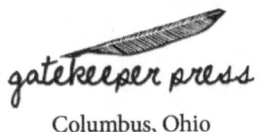

gatekeeper press
Columbus, Ohio

CONTENTS

Chapter 1	Defining the Trust Problem	7
Chapter 2	Institutional Gold Standard in Primary Health Care	13
Chapter 3	Individual Gold Standard in Primary Health Care	17
Chapter 4	Greed	24
Chapter 5	Impairment	33
Chapter 6	Educational Deficiency	41
Chapter 7	Malpractice and Defensive Medicine	50
Chapter 8	Poor Communication	58
Chapter 9	Physician Arrogance	64
Chapter 10	Role of the Patient in the Relationship of Trust	68
Chapter 11	Will Americans Be Able to Afford Health Care in the 21st Century?	75
Chapter 12	What Is Causing the High Cost of Health Care?	78
Chapter 13	The Lack of Consumerism in Health Care	83
Chapter 14	The Role of Overuse in the Misallocation of Healthcare Resources	92
Chapter 15	The Role of Underuse in the Misallocation of Healthcare Resources	104
Chapter 16	Strategies for Coping with High Healthcare Costs	115
Bibliography		125

CHAPTER 1

Defining the Trust Problem

Can *you* trust *your* doctor? Most people receiving health care in the United States today would be correct in saying yes. However, the remaining minority are receiving substandard care from healthcare providers in whom trust is unwarranted and misplaced. This minority translates into a very large number of people at risk. The harm to these individuals and their families from substandard care may be profound and lasting and can occur on multiple levels, including physical, mental, emotional, and financial.

To compound the problem, the average American is confused by the complex process of billing and payment for healthcare services, even when obtaining these services from an ethical provider. As a result, people are commonly overcharged for services that in some cases are not truly necessary or based on scientific evidence. The three primary goals of this book are to shine a light on these important issues by:

- Explaining in detail the scope of the trust problem

- Providing the reader with information that may be used to evaluate a healthcare provider for trustworthiness
- Helping the average healthcare consumer have a better understanding of medical economics.

All with the ultimate aim of helping people use this knowledge to negotiate with ethical healthcare providers to attain high quality, evidenced-based care at a reasonable cost.

This information is especially needed in a time when the United States is facing a crisis in regard to healthcare access and affordability. A rapidly aging American society is creating an unprecedented demand for healthcare services, while a simultaneous shortage of physicians is predicted to get much worse. This makes it all the more important for individuals to be highly informed and proactive healthcare consumers.

The content of this book is based upon our professional and personal experiences as board-certified family practitioners practicing in the same community for over forty years. In addition, we have spent the last three years extensively researching every aspect of the topics covered in the following chapters. Even though the book contains a large degree of harsh criticism for certain members of the medical profession, this is not a kiss-and-tell tale. To the contrary, we have the highest regard for the majority of our colleagues and the work that they do and are honored to have had the privilege to have worked alongside them. We trust that this book will reflect that respect, while also giving an accurate accounting of current problems in our profession that need attention and correction.

When it comes to shopping for a house, automobile, appliance, or an electronic device, American consumers conduct extensive research on products and companies. They comparison shop and acquire a good understanding of the difference between the price and value of a product or service. However, when it comes to health care, these skills commonly disappear. There are many understandable reasons for this. Foremost is the intensely personal, intimate, and sometimes fearful aspect of obtaining health care, as compared to other consumer items and services. Compounding this is the tradition of placing doctors on a pedestal and accepting their healthcare recommendations without question. Being uninformed as a consumer of any product or service can have harmful results, but the personal and financial stakes are much higher and the risks much greater when it comes to health care.

Fortunately, most practicing physicians in this country understand the awesome responsibility that accompanies the privilege of holding a license to practice medicine. They train for many years and work diligently to earn the trust and confidence of the patients they serve. At a minimum, a trustworthy physician must have an excellent basic medical education, outstanding ethics, good communication skills, and a commitment to remain current through continuing medical education. Such physicians do not develop a "God complex" and reject the outdated autocratic approach to healthcare delivery. They view the doctor-patient relationship as a partnership based on shared decision-making. The health care patients receive from physicians with this mentality is generally high quality, accessible, and affordable.

Physicians are, of course, not immune to common human weaknesses and frailties. The characteristics of an untrustworthy doctor are the exact opposite of those described above. Factors leading to untrustworthiness include:

- Incompetence caused by an inferior basic medical education
- Lack of continuing medical education
- Fraud (no valid license or medical degree at all)
- Greed
- Inordinate fear of malpractice

- Arrogance
- Chemical dependency or other incapacitating untreated physical or mental illness.

Such practitioners fall short of even the minimal professional and ethical standards and public expectations.

There are over 800,000 licensed physicians in the United States, and the percentage of those that are untrustworthy is indeed small. However, considering that even one such physician may be providing substandard health care to hundreds or even thousands of individuals, the real and potential harm is substantial. It can be difficult to identify and avoid these untrustworthy physicians.

However, acquiring an awareness of the warning signs is a major step toward becoming a more discerning, sophisticated, and safe healthcare consumer. The ancient Hippocratic Oath is somewhat lengthy and has had multiple interpretations over the years. However, the following is a good synopsis:

> *The regimen I adopt shall be for the benefit of my patients according to my best ability and judgment, and not for their hurt or any wrong. Whatsoever house I enter, there will I go for the benefit of the sick, refraining from all wrongdoing or corruption, and especially from any act of seduction, male or female. May I be favored by God (sic) if the Oath is kept and punished if it is not kept.*

The Hippocratic Oath remains an excellent template for assessing ethical behavior in healthcare providers. A simple definition of ethics is the branch of philosophy that involves defining, defending, and recommending the concepts of right and wrong conduct.

"Wrong conduct" among healthcare providers includes:

- Unprofessional behavior
- Unethical behavior
- Impaired behavior
- Negligent behavior (malpractice)
- Criminal behavior.

These behaviors may occur individually or in combination. For instance, criminal behavior in health care is also unprofessional and unethical. However, all these violate the core of the Hippocratic Oath of *"primum non nocere"* or *"first, do no harm."*

The next two chapters will explore the gold standard for trustworthy healthcare institutions and providers. Subsequent chapters will discuss the warning signs that will let you know a healthcare provider is untrustworthy. Patients equipped with this information will have a comprehensive blueprint for developing a trusting doctor-patient relationship, thereby safeguarding their health.

The final chapters of this book will demonstrate how this partnership with your trusted healthcare provider plays a key role in medical economics. This information will help ensure you're in a position to receive good value for the healthcare services you will purchase throughout your lifetime.

We hope that by implementing the information and advice in this book, you can be part of an overdue solution to this major societal problem. At the very least, this information can help you to attain high-quality health care at a fair and affordable cost, even in the current unsettled medical economic environment.

A mini-glossary

Although a glossary typically appears at the end of a book, we felt the need to include a brief one at this point to clarify and expand upon the terms "doctor/physician" and "patient."

Doctor/Physician: Even though most of the material in this book relates to our occupations as family practitioners, the issues and information discussed in the following material apply to virtually all licensed healthcare providers, not just physicians. This includes medical doctors, nurse practitioners, physician assistants, physical therapists, psychologists, podiatrists, dietitians, etc. So, any reference to "doctor/physician" in this book, unless otherwise specified, is a generic reference to all healthcare providers.

Patient: The term "patient" is not a completely appropriate term for a person receiving health care. The word "patient" derives from the Latin word "patiens," meaning "sufferer." A more comprehensive and inclusive term is "healthcare consumer," and this term will be used interchangeably with "patient" in this book.

CHAPTER 2

Institutional Gold Standard in Primary Health Care

A person's ability to recognize and avoid the perils of substandard health care can be improved with an understanding of what constitutes high-quality health care. The next two chapters will explore in detail the institutional and individual gold standards for healthcare delivery in the primary care setting. The template used for the institutional gold standard component will be the "Patient Centered Medical Home" (PCMH) model.

The origin of the PCMH model can be traced back several decades to the American Academy of Pediatrics. As medical care for children became more advanced and complex due to technological advancement, specialization, and subspecialization, pediatricians recognized that it would be beneficial to have a "medical home" for each child. This medical home would generally be the office of the child's pediatrician or primary care provider.

In the PCMH model, the child receives comprehensive primary medical care from his or her pediatrician. This includes preventive care and treatment for most common childhood illnesses or injuries. In addition, the pediatrician coordinates and monitors all other aspects of the child's care from other healthcare encounters (specialists, subspecialists, pharmacists, outpatient testing and procedures, hospitalizations, etc.). This coordination prevents the potentially confusing and hazardous consequences of fragmented and uncoordinated health care.

Over time, this PCMH concept has grown to include all primary care providers. It is now a formalized program with specific requirements that earn varying degrees of certification. The five main principles of PCMH are:

- Patient-centered: A partnership among practitioners, patients, and their families ensures that decisions respect a patient's wants, needs, and preferences, and that patients have the education and support they need to make decisions and participate in their own care.
- Comprehensive: A team of care providers is wholly accountable for a patient's physical and mental healthcare needs, including prevention and wellness, acute care, and chronic care. Depending on the patient's individual needs, the team may include a small or very large number of healthcare providers and resources.
- Coordinated: Care is organized across all elements of the broader healthcare system, including specialty care, hospitals, home health care, community services, and support.
- Accessible: Patients can access services with shorter waiting times, after-hours care, and 24/7 computer or telephone access.

- Committed to quality and safety: Clinicians and staff enhance quality improvements to ensure that patients and families make informed decisions about their health.[1]

Following these PCMH principles promotes high-quality care in an era of increasing complexity in healthcare delivery. It offers the healthcare consumer a resource for coordination of care that is not always possible in the traditional primary care setting. A lack of this kind of coordination, resulting in fragmented health care, has many potential dangers.

The danger arising from uncoordinated, fragmented care is illustrated when a patient receives prescription medications from multiple doctors. Although physicians should routinely inquire in detail about each patient's current medication and drug allergy history before writing a prescription, all too often this is not the case. In the PCMH model, the primary physician will make every effort to be aware of any changes. This is done by performing a thorough prescription review, also known as a "medication reconciliation," at every patient encounter to be certain there are no avoidable drug interactions or duplications.

Another example of potential danger from uncoordinated health care is a patient receiving care from a specialist who orders a test or procedure that may have already been done. Again, in a perfect world, the specialist would have discovered this in advance by taking a thorough patient history. However, this inappropriate duplication is far too common. In a properly functioning PCMH, the primary physician would prevent this by communicating all relevant information to the specialist in advance. This requires the primary physician

---

1 "Defining the PCMH Home Resource Center." Agency for Healthcare Research and Quality. https://pcmh.ahrq.gov/page/defining-pcmh.

to be aware of the patient's upcoming visit with the specialist, which necessitates the aforementioned thorough history.

The PCMH is a wonderful concept and is a true advancement in primary health care. However, complying with the requirements for official PCMH certification is a complex and expensive effort. Consequently, it has primarily been formally adopted by larger group practices that have the necessary financial and administrative resources required. Smaller solo and group practices (such as ours in rural Texas) are hard-pressed to devote the enormous, uncompensated effort to attain certification.

However, even the smallest primary practice can still implement the PCMH principles, even if it cannot obtain the actual certification. In addition, while the PCMH is the gold standard for primary healthcare delivery, the core principles of placing patients first and at the center of all decisions regarding their health should be applied in every sector of health care.

CHAPTER 3

Individual Gold Standard in Primary Health Care

The previous chapter discussed how a primary care medical clinic can provide evidence of quality and competency in healthcare delivery by attaining PCMH certification or, at a minimum, adhering to the PCMH guidelines. There are equivalent quality and competency indicators for primary care physicians. These include:

- Maintaining an unrestricted medical license
- Attaining and maintaining board certification, which requires consistent continuing medical education
- Active membership in local, state, and national medical societies
- Absence of "red flags" such as an unusual number of malpractice actions
- Transparency with patients regarding referrals to any facility in which a primary care physician may have a financial interest.

With the proper resources, it is not difficult for a healthcare consumer to carry out a thorough background check on both healthcare professionals (physicians, nurse practitioners, physical therapists, psychologists, etc.) and healthcare institutions (clinics, hospitals, clinical laboratories, imaging facilities). Ideally, this background check should occur prior to the initial encounter with a medical practitioner or facility. However, it is still advisable to carry out this background check on a provider or facility with whom you may have a current relationship. Reliable and unbiased resources for performing a background check for proper credentials, malpractice history, and criminal past are widely available on the internet. These include:

- A state's board of medical examiners can provide information on physicians
- The Federation of State Medical Boards (www.FSMB.org) can be used to find the medical board in a given state
- The American Board of Medical Specialties can verify a physician's board certification (https://www.abms.org/verify-certification/).

Similar professional and government internet sites are available for other categories of healthcare providers and some healthcare institutions. This requires searching for the organization that provides the licensing and/or board certification for the specific healthcare category in your state (such as the state board of nursing examiners for nurses, etc.)

Performing a criminal background check on a healthcare provider is more difficult but is nevertheless important to consider. If you need an incentive for this, you should be aware that, according to the Federation of State Medical Boards, as of January 2018 there were eight states that do not require criminal background checks on physicians as a requirement for state licensure (web address above). You should contact your local law enforcement agency of choice to ask for a reliable resource to request a criminal background check. The fees for this range from $25-50, but considering what is at stake this is a reasonable price.

It is very important to point out that using the many unreliable internet resources to assess quality and competency can be misleading and even dangerous. Many internet sites are owned or funded directly or indirectly by the institutions and/or providers that are being recommended on the site. This raises serious concerns about the reliability and bias of these recommendations. There is no foolproof way to avoid an unreliable web resource, but these are some points to consider when assessing a medical internet site:

- Generally, sites with the suffixes .edu and .gov are more likely to be unbiased and reliable. Some examples of reliable sites are:

    — The Center for Disease Control and Prevention - www.CDC.gov
    — The National Institutes of Health - www.NIH.gov

- Well-respected institutions' websites are also generally reliable and include:

    — The Mayo Clinic - www.Mayoclinic.org
    — The Cleveland Clinic - www.my.cleveland-clinic.org

- Some red flags that raise concerns that a website is unreliable include:

    — A large amount of advertising

- Quick and easy solutions to complex and serious health issues
- Promises of miracle cures.

For many individuals, the concept of modern healthcare delivery conjures up high-tech images of a bustling surgical suite, a frantic emergency room, or a patient slowly entering the mysterious cavern of an MRI machine. However, most everyday healthcare encounters occur one-on-one in the private offices of primary care healthcare providers. These providers must, of course, possess up-to-date medical knowledge, good ethics, critical reasoning ability, and sound judgment. However, these qualifications may be of little use to a patient/healthcare consumer in the absence of a good bedside manner.

Most background and credential checking can occur remotely and anonymously. However, bedside manner is the one critical trait of a trustworthy physician that can only be assessed face-to-face, regardless of credentials or certificates.

Bedside manner significantly affects the critical process of communication in a doctor-patient encounter. This includes how the patient is able to express his or her information in the form of symptoms, concerns, or general information to the provider. Likewise, bedside manner affects how a healthcare provider communicates recommendations to the patient in a way that is both understandable and practical to implement. In short, bedside manner is a major factor in how the art of medical practice ensures the science of medicine is of maximum benefit for the patient. Indeed, in some cases, the "art" alone is sufficient without having to involve the "science."

A good bedside manner hinges on the ability of the physician to establish rapport with the patient. Rapport signifies a friendly and harmonious relationship based upon mutual trust and understanding. This requires a cooperative effort in which both parties must communicate effectively. However, this presents a challenge on several levels.

To begin with, society has traditionally conferred an elevated status upon medical practitioners, and this can create an unlevel social playing field, to the disadvantage of the patient. Secondly, the patient often enters a medical encounter with apprehension, or even fear, about the symptoms prompting the encounter. This may be compounded by a person's reluctance or embarrassment about openly discussing intensely personal or emotional matters with a virtual stranger. Therefore, if rapport is to be established, it falls primarily upon the healthcare provider to level the playing field.

This process begins with some very simple interpersonal courtesies such as a warm and sincere introduction from the physician with good eye contact and appropriate body language. There should be an atmosphere of calmness, with no appearance of being impatient or rushed. The medical practitioner generally takes the lead with the conversation, beginning with the reason for the visit. However, the patient must feel the freedom to speak openly and frankly and feel that the practitioner is a good listener. The conversation should be free of complicated medical terminology and jargon ("medical-ese"), conducted at the literacy level of the patient (a later chapter deals in detail with issues of communication).

The following example of a typical first visit in a primary care clinic may help to demonstrate how a good bedside manner can put a patient at ease and markedly reduce stress and anxiety:

The first visit in a primary care office begins with the patient filling out forms detailing personal and family medical history and social history (marital status, education, employment, cultural specifics, etc.). It is appropriate for the practitioner to review this information with the patient before proceeding to the reason for the visit. The patient should be prompted to confirm, clarify, or expand on any information as needed. This is not only proper healthcare technique, but also signals to the patient that the provider has taken the time to review the paperwork and has a basic knowledge of its content.

The basic components of the face-to-face portion of a primary care encounter include taking a thorough history of the reason for the visit, conducting a physical exam, and obtaining any appropriate medical testing (lab, electrocardiogram, imaging). This process should lead to a medical assessment from the provider. This assessment may be a definitive diagnosis in a straightforward case, or a list of diagnostic possibilities if the condition needs further evaluation.

The encounter should conclude with a plan of action for the patient. This may be as simple as reassurance if the condition is minor and will resolve without further intervention or treatment. At the other end of the spectrum with a complex condition, the plan may be quite extensive and include medication, surgery, referrals to specialists, or additional advanced diagnostic testing. A majority of encounters will fall somewhere in between.

Regardless of the simplicity or complexity of the visit, it is imperative that the patient proceed through each phase of the encounter with trust and confidence in the provider. Fortunately, that is the case for most doctor-patient relationships in the United States. This is testimony to the fact that most healthcare providers in the United States have an appropriate bedside manner in addition to possessing other professional and personal attributes that translate into trustworthiness.

So statistically speaking, a patient in the American healthcare system has a very good chance of finding a trustworthy physician with a good bedside manner even when choosing completely at random. However, as the following chapters will reveal, there are serious consequences if that random choice falls upon one of the bad apples in the healthcare profession. Therefore, it is the goal of this book to encourage every healthcare consumer not to choose a provider at random, but to be aware of the potential dangers and take the relatively small amount of time required to do the background checking previously described. However, even when that background check is favorable, there are too many choices of healthcare providers who have good background checks to accept one that does not also possess the vitally important attribute of an excellent bedside manner.

CHAPTER 4

Greed

The previous two chapters discussed the individual and institutional gold standards in primary healthcare delivery. This description will serve as the baseline for the next five chapters that will explore personal traits and characteristics that produce deviations from that standard of excellence in healthcare providers. Among all the negative provider traits and characteristics that contribute to substandard care, greed may be the worst.

Greed may be defined as an insatiable desire to acquire wealth, status, or power. This is particularly inexcusable for doctors in the United States, where physician financial compensation is high. In addition, the public has traditionally bestowed great prestige and privilege upon doctors, resulting in a large degree of personal career satisfaction.

For most physicians, these legitimate professional and financial rewards are more than satisfactory. However, for some, the taste of wealth, status, and power seems to create a ravenous appetite that is satisfied only by coveting more. These individuals are willing to disgrace their profession and their own integrity and humanity in the process. They are apparently oblivious to the fact that, when their activities are exposed, they will endure the disgrace and humiliation of very public legal proceedings. Such disreputable providers are undeterred by the prospect of the loss of a medical license, fines, and even incarceration.

The examples at the end of this chapter are just a few of the hundreds of such cases each year that authorities have identified, prosecuted, and convicted. The actual number of physicians involved in unethical and illegal greed-motivated behavior, and not yet discovered and brought to justice, is obviously much greater. Most of these cases involve nonviolent crimes related to medical practice, but there is a small number that involve assault, rape, and even murder.

Both patients and society as a whole are impacted by this greed. This damage can occur on multiple levels, including physical, psychological, and financial. The most obvious and immediate harm to the patient is financial. A typical example of this involves a provider billing a patient, or the patient's health insurance company, for services that were never actually performed. Although the insurance carrier will generally notify the patient of such billing with an "explanation of benefits" (EOB), these forms are often difficult to interpret, and the patient may not recognize this fraud. Also, the unscrupulous healthcare provider may convince the patient that the "phantom" service actually did occur by providing fictitious results. If the patient has good insurance, the negative financial impact may not be immediately apparent. In a later chapter we will further discuss patient awareness and responsibility in this important area of medical economics.

Another tactic of a greedy healthcare provider involves ordering tests or procedures that are not medically necessary and directing the patient to use facilities or equipment in which the provider has an investment and therefore benefits financially. This is known as self-referral. There are laws on the books that criminalize this activity, but the greedy are willing to take the risk. The amount of money involved is enormous, and detection and enforcement are difficult.

As many of these unnecessary tests and services are complex and highly technological in nature (MRIs, CAT scans, etc.), the costs nationwide are estimated to be in the billions. In addition to the unethical and illegal aspects of this activity, it markedly aggravates the current crisis of the rising costs and limited access to medical services for patients with legitimate healthcare needs.

Beyond the financial harm from this behavior is the risk of physical and psychological harm. Many of the unwarranted tests and procedures ordered by providers motivated by greed come with the possibility of dangerous, potentially life-threatening complications. These complications may be immediate, long-range, or both in nature.

A CAT scan is an example of a test with these potential problems. When this test is performed with an injected or ingested contrast material, it carries the immediate risk of complications from an allergic reaction. In addition, a CAT scan produces significant radiation and can contribute to an increase in future cancer risk. Compounding these problems, there can be "false-positive" results of these unnecessary services that lead to further needless tests. These tests may themselves then result in further complications. Of course, the risks of a truly medically necessary CAT scan are outweighed by the potential benefits when used appropriately, but tragic and avoidable complications may result when not.

Psychological stress for a patient normally accompanies many aspects of even the highest quality health care. This often begins prior to the first encounter with a healthcare professional. When a patient experiences a new symptom, the first thing that frequently occurs is the patient feels apprehension or dread as to whether the symptoms are serious. This leads to additional worry in deciding when or if to seek medical care. So, by the time of the first healthcare encounter, the level of psychological stress may already be very high.

An experienced, trustworthy healthcare provider understands a patient's mindset and will make every effort to calm this anxiety such as by providing reassurance that the symptom or symptoms may represent a minor or manageable condition. However, even if the symptoms do indicate a serious problem, a patient's anxiety can still be lessened by a provider who exhibits understanding and compassion.

In contrast, a greed-motivated physician can prey on people's anxiety. A fearful and apprehensive patient is especially vulnerable and less likely to question recommendations. Indeed, such a patient may unwittingly consider a large degree of advanced imaging and testing to be a sign of thoroughness by an untrustworthy provider. This belief may be furthered by the provider suggesting that the recommended tests and procedures are urgent, warning the patient that delaying may result in major complications.

Even in the best-case scenario, when a patient is not physically harmed as the result of having undergone unnecessary testing, there is almost always psychological harm arising from the increased anxiety of the testing process and waiting anxiously for results.

A common example would be a patient with chest pain who presents to his doctor with an understandable fear that his symptoms may represent heart disease. When managed by a responsible healthcare provider, a through history, physical exam, and a few noninvasive and relatively inexpensive tests may show that heart disease is not the cause of the chest pain. Conversely, an unethical physician with a financial interest in a facility that performs advanced cardiac testing may convince the patient to undergo an invasive cardiac catheterization "just to be sure."

While most individuals complete this procedure without harm, a few will suffer serious complications that include a stroke. Whether or not the patient escapes without serious harm, there is no escaping the psychological stress for both the patients and their family and friends as this process unfolds.

Although the blame for this shameful situation rests squarely on the unprincipled healthcare provider, patients can unwittingly contribute to the problem. It is human nature to be awed by high-tech medical marvels such as MRIs, CT scans, cardiac catherization, etc. If a patient has a troublesome symptom such as chest pain, it is normal to be apprehensive and want to obtain an accurate and rapid diagnosis. A patient may feel pressured to accept almost any intervention recommended.

In this era of ever-increasing health insurance costs, it is also human nature for a patient to feel "I must get my money's worth" from expensive healthcare premium payments. Yet this is not a wise decision and can play into the hands of an unscrupulous healthcare provider. More details on the role and responsibility of the patient in health care are discussed in a later chapter.

The percentage of doctors involved in these types of unethical activities is small. However, as the following examples indicate, such doctors aren't rare, and the impact can be far-reaching and have devastating consequences to patients involved:

- In Baytown, Texas, two married physicians were sentenced in April 2010 for defrauding Medicare, Medicaid, and more than a dozen private insurers. They pleaded guilty to conspiracy to commit healthcare and mail fraud as well as one count of healthcare fraud for their decade-long scam of billing healthcare providers for injection procedures that they did not perform. U.S. District Judge David Hittner sentenced them to 15 and eight years in federal prison, respectively. A restitution order of more than $40 million was imposed.[2]

---

2   "Local Physicians Sentenced Again – Must Pay More Than $37 Million In Restitution." Department of Justice.

- A Houston doctor was sentenced to three and a half years in federal prison for fraudulently billing Medicare and Medicaid for hundreds of thousands of dollars in treatment and tests that patients didn't need or receive.[3]
- In 2016, the federal government announced an unprecedented nationwide sweep led by the Medicare Fraud Strike Force (a multi-agency team of U.S. federal, state, and local investigators that target Medicare fraud and abuse) in 36 federal districts, resulting in criminal and civil charges against 301 individuals, including 61 doctors, nurses, and other licensed medical professionals, for their alleged participation in healthcare fraud schemes involving approximately $900 million in false billings.[4]
- Every year the Office of the Inspector General in the U.S. Department of Health and Human Services successfully convicts hundreds of individuals and businesses for Medicare fraud. These cases involve billions of dollars in losses that are borne by the taxpayer.[5]

Last modified April 30, 2015. https://www.justice.gov/usao-sdtx/pr/local-physicians-sentenced-again-must-pay-more-37-million-restitution.

3 Banks, Gabrielle. "Houston Doctor Sentenced to Prison for Medicare Fraud." Houston Chronicle, March 24, 2016. https://www.houstonchronicle.com/news/houston-texas/houston/article/Houston-doctor-sentenced-to-prison-for-Medicare-7045012.php.

4 "Medicare Fraud Strike Force." U.S. Department of Health and Human Services. https://oig.hhs.gov/fraud/strike-force/.

5 "Criminal and Civil Enforcement." U.S. Department of Health and Human Services.https://oig.hhs.gov/fraud/enforcement/criminal/.

The above are examples of criminal behavior by physicians and other healthcare providers that are committed in the course of their roles in healthcare delivery. These make up a large percentage of felony convictions in healthcare providers, but the following cases involved violent criminal behavior, including assault, murder, and rape.

- An admitted physician serial killer is currently serving life in prison without the possibility of parole for murdering four persons. Authorities suspect he was involved in as many as 60 fatal poisonings of patients, colleagues, and family. His story has been featured in the Investigation Discovery Channel series "*Untouchables*."[6]
- A Montgomery, Alabama, physician surrendered his license for administering fake flu vaccines in 2005. In 2013, this same doctor was convicted in a murder-for-hire plot.[7,8]
- In 1996, the state of Maryland licensed a physician who had pleaded guilty to raping a woman at gunpoint.[9]
- In 2004, a Veterans Administration hospital hired a psychiatrist with known felony convictions. A

---

6 "Dr. Joseph Michael Swango." Murderpedia. https://murderpedia.org/male.S/s/swango-michael.htm.

7 Bullock, Mark. "Doctor Confesses to Faking Flu Shots." WSFA. Last modified July 27, 2005. https://www.wsfa.com/story/4236706/doctor-confesses-to-faking-flu-shots/.

8 Andrist, Eric. "Dr. Zev-David Nash." The Patient Safety League. Last modified November , 2015. http://4patientsafety.org/2015/11/03/dr-zev-david-nash/.

9 Lowes, Robert. "Medical Board Faulted for Licensing Convicted Rapist." Medscape. Last modified November 25, 2014. https://www.medscape.com/viewarticle/835430.

year after the hire, a criminal check revealed eight arrests including burglary, reckless driving resulting in death, and drug dealing.[10]

- A New York gynecologist was charged with first-degree assault for carving his initials into the abdomen of a woman who had just delivered a child by caesarean section.[11]
- A Colorado optometrist was accused of sexually molesting a seven-year-old during an exam in 2006. The allegation was swept under the rug until he assaulted a four-year-old in 2011. Only then did he lose his license.[12]

In most instances, a felony conviction will prevent a physician from maintaining a license to practice medicine. However, there are exceptions. This issue is generally regulated at the state level. Each state medical board is independent and the strictness or leniency in this matter can vary greatly. The majority of state medical boards currently do a criminal background check in the process of issuing physician medical licenses, and this information is available to the

---

10 Slack, Donovan. "USA TODAY Investigation: VA Knowingly Hires Doctors with Past Malpractice Claims, Discipline for Poor Care." USA Today, December 3, 2017. https://www.usatoday.com/story/news/politics/2017/12/03/usa-today-investigation-va-knowingly-hires-doctors-past-malpractice-claims-discipline-poor-care/909170001/.

11 Steinhauer, Jennifer. "Patient Settles Case Of Initials Cut in Skin." New York Times, February 12, 2000. https://www.nytimes.com/2000/02/12/nyregion/patient-settles-case-of-initials-cut-in-skin.html.

12 Gladstone, Jennifer. "Medical Background Checks Lacking." Ebi. Last modified September 28, 2016. https://www.ebiinc.com/resources/blog/medical-background-checks-lacking.

public in addition to information on education, malpractice, and non-criminal disciplinary actions.

However, as noted previously, there are still some states in which state medical boards do not routinely perform criminal background checks (see chapter 3). Also, individual state laws vary widely regarding the rights of convicted felons. Thus, even though the risk of healthcare consumers encountering a convicted felon as their chosen healthcare provider is not great, it is prudent to take the simple and relatively inexpensive steps to do a basic criminal background check on any existing or potential provider.

CHAPTER 5

Impairment

The delivery of high-quality health care is severely compromised if a provider's judgment is impaired by any physical or mental health condition. This issue may develop from a wide range of conditions, and most of these are difficult to recognize unless very severe or advanced. Though the most common forms of healthcare provider impairment include alcohol or drug abuse or dependency, there are many other serious medical and psychological disorders that are also of great concern if not successfully recognized and treated. These include dementia, depression, gambling addiction, sexual addiction, and post-traumatic stress disorder. Even more subtle situations, such as a serious physical illness, the death of a family member, divorce, financial problems, legal entanglements, excessive fatigue, and professional burnout can weaken a provider's judgment and performance.

Accurate statistics on drug dependency and other impairment conditions are difficult to obtain. One obvious reason for this is that providers currently or formally afflicted may be reluctant to provide truthful and complete information about their current or past problems. Studies surveying healthcare professionals indicate rates of alcohol and other drug addiction as high as 15 percent.[13] Data on the causes of impairment other than chemical dependency is more difficult to quantify. Nevertheless, the overall issue of healthcare provider impairment is significant.[14]

There are factors that may contribute to a higher-than-average rate of chemical dependency specifically among physicians. This includes a highly competitive and intense academic process that typically begins at a very young age and lasts many years into early adulthood. During this process, prospective healthcare providers are exposed to illness, injury, and death at an age much younger than most of their non-medical contemporaries. Healthcare providers also have easy access to highly addictive pharmaceuticals.

These factors in no way constitute an excuse for abusing and becoming dependent on alcohol or other substances. Indeed, most physicians deal with the pressures of life and live sober and unimpaired lives. However, just as within the general population, a minority of physicians will find themselves chemically dependent or otherwise impaired.

When faced with addiction or other impairments, there is a natural human tendency for the affected individual to try to prevent the condition from becoming public knowledge. Addicted individuals also commonly minimize, or deny, their problem. Since physicians are granted elevated social status, prestige, and financial security, this pressure to avoid discovery is heightened. In addition, the practitioner's family, and

---

13 Berge, Keith H., Marvin D. Seppala, and Agnes M. Schipper. "Chemical Dependency and the Physician." Mayo Clinic Proceedings 84, no. 7 (July 2009): 625-31. https://doi.org/10.1016/S0025-6196(11)60751-9

14 "The Scope of Physician Addiction." Physician Health Program. https://www.physicianhealthprogram.com/scope-physician-addiction/.

even professional colleagues, often try to shield him or her from exposure. All this denial and deception serves only to delay the recognition, acceptance, and intervention that are so vitally necessary for recovery. Even more troublesome is that any delay in detection and treatment leaves the unsuspecting patients of the impaired physician at serious risk.

Defining the magnitude of this potential danger for patients is difficult. As noted above, the rate of chemical dependency for physicians is in the 8-15 percent range. Taking the low end of 8 percent and applying this to the almost 900,000 practicing physicians in the United States, this equates to over 70,000 impaired doctors (over 130,000 if using the high end of 15 percent). This does not include those physicians with other conditions that adversely affect judgment as mentioned above (dementia, untreated depression, burnout, gambling addiction, etc.).

In addition to these very large numbers of afflicted physicians, there will be large numbers of impaired individuals among the millions of other healthcare professionals. Each of these can also inflict harm if their judgment is impaired. There are several hundred thousand nurse practitioners and physician assistants practicing in the United States. Physical therapists number over 200,000. There are four million licensed nurses (3.3 million RNs and over 800,000 LPNs). When you include pharmacists, psychologists, and dentists, the total number is in excess of five million. The rate of impairment in all these groups can logically be assumed to be at least that of the general population.

These staggering numbers are scary, but they do not mean that every impaired healthcare professional is harming every patient encountered. Many of these providers will be in the very early stages of their condition, when their judgment may not be markedly diminished. If they are making medical recommendations for routine or minor conditions, the risk to patients is likely small. However, any such preventable risk, no matter how small, should be considered unacceptable.

Some impaired healthcare providers recognize their condition and suspend practice and seek treatment. Others are identified by law enforcement or professional societies and are temporarily or permanently removed from medical practice. If there is any good news to this issue, it is that the prognosis is often favorable for addicted practitioners that commit to effective treatment programs. Also, most severe depression and burnout can be successfully treated.

Unfortunately, there are circumstances in which there is little chance of recovery. These include those chemically or otherwise addicted individuals who remain in denial, refuse treatment, or fail to respond to recovery programs. There are some neurological conditions, such as most types of dementia, for which there is no treatment that would permit a return to practice. There are also some impaired providers who are successfully treated but choose to retire or enter another line of work. This is especially common with those experiencing severe burnout.

Of course, the impaired providers posing the greatest threat to patients are those that remain undetected and untreated. The greater the degree of impairment and loss of judgment, the greater the risk to the patients these providers encounter. As some of the following cases will demonstrate, the results of the actions of even one seriously impaired healthcare provider can create serious physical and psychological damage to thousands of patients:

- Nearly 8,000 people in eight states needed hepatitis tests after an itinerant hospital technician was caught injecting himself with patients' pain medicine and refilling the syringes with saline. He infected at least 46 persons with hepatitis, mostly in New Hampshire. This activity is called "drug diversion."[15]

- Fifty-five women contracted hepatitis C after having abortions performed between 2008 and 2009 by an anesthetist with a drug dependence. He was prosecuted for infecting these women while in his care.[16]
- A Colorado surgical technologist infected hospital patients with hepatitis in 2008 and 2009 by injecting herself with fentanyl and leaving behind dirty needles.[17]
- A neurosurgeon was sentenced to life in prison in 2017 for assault with a deadly weapon (described as his hands and surgical instruments). Records indicate a number of surgeries resulting in both death and maiming of patients. This occurred over several years and in multiple hospitals before his medical license was revoked. Suspected of being under the influence of cocaine while operating during the fourth year of his surgical residency, he was sent for treatment but was then allowed to return to his

---

15   Eisler, Peter. "Doctors, Medical Staff on Drugs Put Patients at Risk." USA Today, April 15, 2014. https://www.usatoday.com/story/news/nation/2014/04/15/doctors-addicted-drugs-healthcare-diversion/7588401/.

16   Schalit, Naomi. "How Was a Drug-addicted Doctor with Hep C Able to Infect His Patients?" Health and Medicine. The Conversation, February 26, 2013. http://theconversation.com/how-was-a-drug-addicted-doctor-with-hep-c-able-to-infect-his-patients-12166.

17   Olinger, David. "Drug-addicted, Dangerous and Licensed for the Operating Room." Denver Post, June 2016. https://www.denverpost.com/2016/04/23/drug-addicted-dangerous-and-licensed-for-the-operating-room/.

- residency program. His case has been featured in the Oxygen cable channel series, *License to Kill*, as well as in a podcast series entitled "Dr. Death," produced by Wondery Media.[18]
- A radiology technician working at the Mayo Clinic in Jacksonville, FL, was sentenced to 30 years in prison on 10 federal charges that included tampering with a consumer product that caused great bodily harm, one resulting in death, and stealing the pain-killer fentanyl.[19]

The above instances are extreme, but there are many more common circumstances occurring daily in healthcare delivery in which patients are potentially at risk. Examples include:

- A surgeon exhausted and suffering from "burnout" operating on patients
- An intoxicated radiologist missing an abnormal finding on an x-ray
- A severely clinically depressed family doctor whose inability to concentrate during a patient encounter results in prescribing a drug to which a patient is allergic
- A nurse who is an active victim of spousal abuse and is understandably preoccupied gives the incorrect medication to a hospital patient.

---

18 "Christopher Duntsch." Wikipedia. Last modified January 2020. https://en.wikipedia.org/wiki/Christopher_Duntsch.

19 "Radiology Technician Sentenced to 30 Years for Product Tampering." The Federal Bureau of Investigation. Last modified September 11, 2012. https://archives.fbi.gov/archives/jacksonville/press-releases/2012/radiology-technician-sentenced-to-30-years-for-product-tampering.

Although virtually everyone would agree that there should be zero tolerance for impaired practitioners being active in healthcare delivery, there are very few proactive safeguards for the public currently in place. Many professions in which public safety is on the line (airline pilots, train and subway engineers, etc.) impose random drug testing, but this is not common in the medical profession. However, this is slowly beginning to change. An example would be among anesthesiologists, who are estimated to comprise 20-30 percent of all chemically dependent physicians. The suspected reasons for this high rate include the close proximity to large quantities of highly addictive drugs and the relative ease of being able to divert these for personal use. Regardless of the reasons, this large percentage in such a high-risk specialty has prompted a number of hospitals and surgical centers to mandate random drug testing in this specialty.

There is growing support to extend this testing to all physicians performing invasive or high-risk procedures, such as surgeons, emergency room physicians, intensive care specialists, interventional cardiologists, and interventional radiologists. It would seem to follow that this should extend to all the other healthcare professionals that assist the specialists in these activities, covering a wide range of nurses and medical technicians.

The logical progression of this movement would be to extend random drug testing (and screening for other types of impairment) to all healthcare professionals whose impaired judgment could harm a patient. That would effectively include virtually all healthcare professionals in active clinical settings. The costs and logistics of such a wide-ranging program are barriers to implementing this type of public safety measure, but other safety-sensitive professions have managed to figure it out. It may take more public outcry and legislative pressure to effect these changes, but the current status quo is unacceptable.

Until, and if, widespread random drug screening (and screening for other forms of impairment) becomes a reality, it behooves each individual healthcare consumer to be aware of this issue and the potential danger it presents. As mentioned in the first paragraph of this chapter, it is often difficult to identify an impaired provider until the condition is advanced. There are, however, personal or behavioral warning signs, or red flags that can be helpful. These include:

- Slurred speech
- Inappropriate comments
- Odor of alcohol or drugs
- Disheveled appearance
- Forgetfulness beyond what is common
- Excessive irritability
- Mood swings
- Frequent rescheduling of appointments or absences from work.

If a healthcare consumer encounters evidence of active healthcare provider impairment, there are several recommended actions to take.

1. Change healthcare providers immediately.
2. Take steps to protect other healthcare consumers that are at risk. This includes speaking to the administrator of the clinic or hospital if available.
3. It's also advisable to notify the medical board or other government agency responsible for oversight of the impaired provider. This notification may be made anonymously if needed.

CHAPTER 6

Educational Deficiency

The education of a trustworthy healthcare provider is a career-long process. The following information applies to physicians, but all healthcare providers are faced with these requirements in varying degrees. There are two educational components involved:

- First, there are the academic and clinical requirements for obtaining a license to legally practice medicine.
- Second, there is continuing medical education (CME), which is equally important and critical to keep pace with changes and advances in medicine.

A deficiency in either of these components will diminish the trustworthiness of a physician.

The typical education to acquire a license to practice medicine as a physician in the United States requires 11 or more years following high school graduation. This includes four years in college, four years in medical school, and three or more years in a residency program. There are required national and/or state board examinations to demonstrate competency before a medical license is issued. In addition, each medical specialty requires passing a specialty board examination and undergoing a periodic recertification process in order to become or remain board certified.

As soon as the physician has completed the long and arduous basic educational requirements described above, the process of CME must start. The importance of this is evident when considering that the information learned in the first years of medical school will be over five to eight years old by the time a physician has concluded a three- to five-year residency program. While much of that material will have remained current and valid, the rapid advances in medicine in this age of high technology guarantees that there will be major changes and advances that must be mastered and incorporated into daily practice. In addition, there will be some practices that were once acceptable that must be discarded. Considering the average physician may practice for 40-50 years, the importance of CME is obvious.

Fortunately, virtually every accredited medical school in the United States meets or exceeds the high standards required for a quality basic education. In addition, the students entering U.S. medical schools come from the top of their college classes. The average GPA for an entering medical school student in the U.S. is above 3.7/4.[20] As a result, it is highly likely that every student who graduates from an accredited U.S. medical school will have a good basic medical education.

---

20   Kowarski, Ilana. "How High of a College GPA Is Needed for Med School?" US News. https://www.usnews.com/education/best-graduate-schools/top-medical-schools/articles/2018-10-02/how-high-of-a-college-gpa-is-necessary-to-get-into-medical-school.

There is a worn-out joke that asks: "What do you call the person who finishes last in his or her medical school class?" The answer: "A doctor." To be certain, the individual who finishes academically at the top of a prestigious Ivy League medical school might rightfully be expected to be more highly qualified than one who finishes at the bottom of a small state medical school. Yet there are exceptions to this assumption, and many of the finest medical practitioners come from medical schools that are not at the top of the prestige list. For the reasons stated above, virtually all U.S.-trained physicians are equipped with the basic academic and clinical tools to become trustworthy practitioners.

There has been some concern about the quality of the basic education of students attending certain foreign medical schools. These include schools in which the quality of the basic science and clinical curricula do not meet the standards of U.S. medical schools. However, not included in this concern are the graduates of many fine foreign medical schools with basic medical educational and clinical standards that are on par with U.S. medical schools. In order to obtain a license to practice medicine in the U.S., every graduate from a foreign medical school is required to have completed some clinical training in an accredited U.S. institution. In addition, graduates must pass examinations that test their basic medical knowledge. These additional safeguards make it unlikely that any person with a substandard medical education will be able to legally practice medicine in this country.

The main concern regarding a deficiency in basic medical education is fraud, which involves practicing medicine without a valid medical license. There are many documented instances of individuals without a medical license and fraudulent credentials presenting themselves to an unsuspecting public as legally licensed physicians. This is a criminal offense and clearly the most dangerous form of "physician" educational deficiency. These are a few examples of this uncommon, but not rare, circumstance:

- A former prison medic who served time for bank robbery set up a medical practice in a small East Texas town where he saw patients for an extended period until he was caught ordering drugs under the name of the real doctor whose name he was using.[21]
- In Tampa, FL, two individuals posing as doctors were arrested for performing liposuction on multiple patients, many of whom had to seek treatment at another medical facility for complications of the procedure; four of these were scarred permanently and suffered severe pain.[22]
- In New York, an investigation of the purchase of several thousand fraudulent medical degrees from the Dominican Republic resulted in the arrest of multiple individuals for practicing medicine with bogus credentials.[23]
- A surgical assistant who posed as a plastic surgeon, performing medical procedures on more than 50

---

21   Derbyshire, Robert C. "The Make-Believe Doctors (1993)." Credential Watch. Last modified February 25, 2005. https://www.credentialwatch.org/inv/impostors.shtml
22   Marrero, Tony. "Victims Disfigured by Unlicensed Town 'N Country Liposuction Center, Authorities Say." Tampa Bay Times, April 1, 2017. https://www.tampabay.com/news/publicsafety/crime/two-charged-with-performing-liposuction-without-license-in-town-n-country/2332261/.
23   Lyons, Richard D. "2 Medical Schools Closed in Scandal." The New York Times, May 16, 1984. https://www.nytimes.com/1984/05/16/us/2-medical-schools-closed-in-scandal.html.

victims was sentenced to six years in prison after pleading guilty to second-degree felony assault, criminal impersonation, and unauthorized practice of a physician.[24]

Although the risk of encountering an individual attempting to practice medicine without a license is small, the potential for physical harm to a healthcare consumer who does unwittingly receive services from a fraudulent practitioner is substantial.

Determining if a physician has a legitimate basic medical school and residency education is a straightforward, one-step procedure. Identifying a deficiency in CME is more complicated, because it is a dynamic and career-long process. There is a certain amount of continuing education that is mandatory in order for a physician to maintain a valid medical license in most states. However, these requirements vary greatly from state to state. As published on the Medscape website, in January 2019, examples of the range of annual general CME requirements for maintenance of state licensure for a physician varied from 50 in Massachusetts to zero in Indiana. In addition to the requirements from the state medical boards, each medical specialty has mandatory requirements to maintain board certification status. These "maintenance of certification" (MOC) CME goals are typically greater than those required to maintain a valid medical license.

There is some objective evidence to suggest that a small percentage of physicians do not engage in enough CME to remain trustworthy. A recent report revealed that approximately 13 percent of physicians fail to meet the current MOC

---

24 Worthington, Danika. "Fake Denver Doctor Who Posed as a Plastic Surgeon Sentenced to 6 Years in Prison." Denver Post, June 2, 2017. https://www.denverpost.com/2017/06/02/denver-fake-plastic-surgeon-sentenced/.

requirements of Internal Medicine. If not corrected, this could lead to the loss of board certification.[25] However, just as with basic medical education, most physicians meet and exceed the minimal CME requirements of state medical boards and specialty organizations.

From the time that a physician enters medical school until the time he or she finishes residency training, there will have already been substantial changes in the "standard of care" and advances in diagnostic and treatment options. This realization makes it abundantly clear to the newly minted physician that it will be impossible to remain competent and trustworthy without a lifetime commitment to high-quality CME. This is true no matter how ethical a physician may be or how great of a bedside manner he or she possesses. However, there is currently a controversy surrounding CME. Some would say it is approaching a crisis.

The area in which the CME controversy is most evident is the MOC process that currently exists for most medical specialties. In summary, the MOC is a process overseen by the American Board of Medical Specialties (ABMS). The ABMS requires that any physicians who have obtained initial board certification in their specialty through an examination after completing their residency must begin and continue a recertification process. This includes significant annual study and performance requirements and a repeat examination every ten years. While this would appear on the surface to be a reasonable approach to ensure that a physician maintains competency in the given specialty, it has come under fire as failing to accomplish its stated goals and being overpriced and bur-

---

[25] Arthur, Gale. "The Onerous Rules of the American Board of Internal Medicine and the National Quality Forum Reward Bureaucrats, Undermine Physician Morale, and Do Not Improve Patient Care." Mo Med 115, no. 4 (July 2018): 316-18. https://www.ncbi.nlm.nih.gov/pmc/articles/PMC6140246/.

densome. There are many who believe the MOC process has evolved, or devolved, to become a bureaucratic boondoggle whose main benefit is to certain highly paid individuals that administer the process.

The major complaint of those physicians who oppose the MOC process is that there is no reliable research or scientific evidence to support that MOC, as it currently exists, accomplishes its laudable goals. In fact, it can be effectively argued that MOC ironically does the opposite, by requiring physicians to engage in activities unproven to enhance the knowledge and skills that they use in daily practice. Critics argue that this is time that could be spent pursing CME that is more relevant and useful.[26]

It is logical to ask how this situation could have been allowed to develop over the years. The answer would seem to be the same as what happens in many organizations (government, education, etc.) when the bureaucratic process creates a top-down environment in which those individuals in decision-making positions have lost contact with the rank and file that they are supposed to serve. This appears to be confirmed in a recent survey of practicing physicians released by the Mayo Clinic that indicates that only 24 percent thought the MOC process was relevant to improving their knowledge and skills and 81 percent considered it burdensome.[27]

---

26   Kaplan, Deborah A. "Physicians' Battle to Limit Maintenance of Certification Requirements Continues Despite Testing Changes." Medical Economics. Last modified October 2018. https://www.medicaleconomics.com/business/physicians-battle-limit-maintenance-certification-requirements-continues-despite-testing-changes.

27   Cook, David A., Morris J. Blachman, Colin P. West, and Christopher M. Wittich. "Physician Attitudes About Maintenance of Certification." Mayo Clinic Proceedings 91,

Almost half of U.S. state legislatures are now considering "Right to Care" legislation that prohibits state medical boards from requiring physicians to comply with MOC to maintain their medical license.[28] Although this is welcomed by most physicians, there is hope that this will also extend to insurance companies and hospitals. Until that occurs, this deficiency may still leave physicians feeling coerced to comply with an MOC process that they believe to be inferior to alternative CME activities. If they do not comply, they may be dropped from the networks of insurance payors and/or lose hospital privileges. The real tragedy is that there is evidence that MOC is one of the major factors that is driving good physicians into early retirement, further worsening the growing problem of access to medical care. It also makes entering medicine less attractive to young qualified students considering which career path to take.

However, as needed reform takes place, it is very important that the necessity of CME not be weakened, and the baby is not thrown out with the bathwater. It would be incorrect to stereotype every individual at the ABMS as an out-of-touch, overpaid bureaucrat who is unsympathetic to the practicing rank-and-file physician that must comply with MOC. No doubt many at the ABMS are highly qualified and well-meaning. In fact, there have been recent changes in the MOC process in response to the growing criticism. However, at the time of this printing, these changes have not satisfied most of the critics of MOC.

---

no. 10 (October 2016): 1336-45. https://doi.org/10.1016/j.mayocp.2016.07.004.

28 Sullivan, Thomas. "Anti-MOC Laws Picking Up Steam Across the United States." Policy Med. Last modified May 4, 2018. https://www.policymed.com/2017/06/anti-moc-laws-picking-up-steam-across-the-united-states.html.

Most thoughtful physicians who are critics and advocates for change in the current MOC process understand that they have a responsibility for a lifetime of continuing medical education. They also are more than willing to demonstrate this to state boards, specialty organizations, and the general public. Their main goal is to promote a system that is streamlined, affordable, and most importantly, truly relevant to the process of keeping a physician current with changes and advances in health care in a particular field of medical practice.

Even physicians with good ethics, an excellent bedside manner, and no issues with greed or impairment can become "untrustworthy" if they do not keep pace with CME. It is possible today for physicians to practice with minimal CME. As noted above, in some states there is no CME requirement to maintain a medical license. There is no magic number of hours spent on CME that will assure maintenance of competency. However, there is no question that significant CME efforts are necessary to keep pace in this current environment of rapid changes and advances. As a point of reference, the American Academy of Family Physicians requires 50 hours of CME per year to maintain membership in the academy. Our experience as family practitioners is that it takes significantly more than 50 hours per year to stay current with medical practices.

It is important that healthcare consumers are certain that their healthcare providers did complete a legitimate basic course of education and are staying current with changes and advances in their fields of practice. As noted in chapter 3, healthcare consumers can use the internet to search the state board of medical examiners in order to verify a physician's basic medical training and acquire some information regarding compliance with CME requirements for maintaining a medical license.

CHAPTER 7

Malpractice and Defensive Medicine

Medical malpractice occurs when a patient is harmed because of an act of negligence by a healthcare provider. This matter goes to the core of trustworthiness in the doctor-patient relationship. There are two major malpractice issues of which every healthcare consumer needs to be aware.

The first is that certain physicians have a record of multiple malpractice lawsuits that may be a cause for concern. A large percentage of providers who have been in practice for some years will have at least one malpractice suit filed against them. Doctors in high-risk specialties (obstetrics, surgery, etc.) may have several. What should create a red flag for a healthcare consumer is a pattern of multiple lawsuits that are settled in favor of the patient filing the suit.

The second problem is an excessive fear of malpractice that can be the source of what is known as "defensive medicine." There is evidence that this problem is widespread among physicians and all healthcare providers. Every physician is, of course, aware of the risk of malpractice. When a physician delivers high-quality care, there is a very low probability of being named in a malpractice suit. However, there are well-documented cases of physicians ending up in court even when delivering the best care possible. As a result, physicians cannot help but be concerned that they could be sued.

One benefit of this concern is that it may produce a "healthy fear" of malpractice. This can become positive motivation to avoid becoming complacent or careless in making decisions that could harm patients. However, if that fear becomes excessive, it can lead to a doctor practicing defensive medicine. This will be described in detail below, and it can clearly cause harm to patients. When this occurs, the trustworthiness of the physician is clearly diminished. This chapter is intended to present a balanced assessment of this complex issue.

Medical malpractice is a tragic situation for the affected patient, who may suffer physical, emotional, and financial damage. It is also one of the most difficult personal issues that a healthcare provider may encounter in his or her professional career. When a malpractice case is filed or goes to court, there will generally be a ruling that favors one side or the other. However, there are no true "winners" in the process, as both parties will typically have endured a long and painful ordeal. In addition, there is strong evidence that the current state of medical malpractice in the U.S. has adverse effects on society in terms of healthcare costs and access.

There can be confusion about what constitutes true medical malpractice versus a bad medical outcome. Medical malpractice is legally defined as occurring when a medical practitioner's action deviates from an accepted "standard of care" and that action then causes harm to a patient. The "standard of care" is *defined* as what a reasonably prudent medical provider would or would not have done under the same or similar circumstances.

By definition, every true medical malpractice event has a bad medical outcome, but not every bad medical outcome is malpractice. These are some examples of actual cases that represent true medical malpractice:

- A surgeon performs an amputation of the wrong limb
- A child suffers brain damage during childbirth due to a lack of accepted fetal monitoring procedures
- A patient suffers permanent hearing damage due to an overdose of an antibiotic as the result of a nurse misreading a physician's handwritten order
- A patient presents to an emergency room with chest pain and is sent home with medication for "indigestion" without a cardiac evaluation and later that night dies from a massive coronary
- A woman mentions a breast lump during a physical exam, but no mammogram or further testing is ordered, and she later is diagnosed with advanced breast cancer
- A patient with leg pain is sent home from an emergency room with pain medication for a "muscle strain" and later develops complications from a blood clot in that leg
- A patient presenting with severe abdominal pain is sent home with a diagnosis of "stomach flu" without blood work or imaging and is later determined to have a ruptured appendix
- A young man presents with a severe "thunderclap" headache and is discharged home with pain medication without imaging and later that day dies from a ruptured cerebral aneurysm.

Each of the above examples are instances where the standard of care was clearly not met. In such cases, the patient or family members are completely justified in seeking compensation through the legal system. This may be settled with a jury trial or out-of-court settlement.

Yet many malpractice actions are filed when there is no negligence. The human body is so very complex that even when the highest standards of medical care are followed, a bad outcome can result. In such instances the patient sustains an injury, or dies, as the result of medical treatment. However, there are situations in which these things occur, and healthcare provider's actions are consistent with the accepted standard of care and not negligence. It is human nature to look for a cause, or someone to blame, for a bad medical outcome. Emotions run very high under these circumstances, and decisions that are made may not always be rational. The result is that the legal system must deal with a large number of cases without true merit, and some of these are truly frivolous. The fact that most malpractice claims that are filed are not true negligence is supported by the statistics of the outcome of cases.

Less than 5 percent of medical malpractice cases ever go to a jury, and those that do are ruled in favor of the physician almost 80 percent of the time. Nine out of ten of all cases are settled out of court, and over 80 percent that are settled do so with no payment to the patient or patient's family.[29]

Whether true negligence or a bad outcome, every malpractice suit that is filed involves mental, emotional, physical, and financial suffering for many individuals. Both the individual filing the suit and the health provider being sued will spend many months, or even years, in a confrontational environment. Whether one party ultimately "wins" or a settlement out-of-court is reached, the process takes a great toll on both parties. In the case of true malpractice or negligence,

---

29   Peters, Philip G. "Twenty Years of Evidence on the Outcomes of Malpractice Claims." Clinical Orthopaedics and Related Research 467, no. 2 (February 2009): 352-57. https://doi.org/10.1007/s11999-008-0631-7.

the person filing the lawsuit will hopefully prevail and feel at least somewhat compensated. In the case of a bad outcome or non-negligence, the defendant physician will hopefully prevail and feel somewhat vindicated. However, a fair and just outcome is not a certainty, and the legal system does get it wrong on both sides. So, as stated above, it is difficult to call anyone a true "winner" in this process.

Another "loser" in this issue is the healthcare system as a whole. One of the very unfortunate consequences associated with medical malpractice is the above-mentioned problem of "defensive medicine." This involves medical practitioners, primarily physicians, taking precautionary, or "defensive" measures to avoid being named in a malpractice suit. This may involve ordering unnecessary tests or procedures or making referrals to minimize the possibility of missing a diagnosis that would create a possible malpractice action. This defensive, and unnecessary, action is most likely to occur with symptoms that could be a sign of a serious or even life-threatening condition such as chest pain, abdominal pain, or headache. It is also more likely to occur when there is no established doctor-patient relationship, such as in an emergency room, but it can happen with any healthcare encounter.

Defensive medicine is unquestionably wasteful and burdensome to a healthcare system that is currently plagued by ever-increasing cost and access problems. More importantly, it can be the source of harm for patients. Very similar to the circumstance covered in the chapter on greed, unnecessary medical tests arising from defensive medicine activity have more potential danger than the obvious financial waste. They carry the same problems of false positive test results, potential serious side effects or complications, and the inevitable emotional strain for the patient and family who must endure the stress of waiting for results of tests that by all rights should never have been recommended.

Defensive medicine is an overall wasteful and potentially dangerous activity. Although it is not truly excusable, it may be better understood if examined in the context of historical changes in society that produced a highly lawsuit-prone environment in which a malpractice crisis developed. Medical malpractice lawsuits in the U.S. date to the late 1700s, but they were relatively uncommon until the 1960s.[30] At this time there was a convergence of medical, legal, and social factors that created a spike in malpractice suits.

Healthcare delivery in the 20th century was becoming much more complex with major advances in diagnostic and therapeutic options. The public embraced these modern medical miracles that were saving lives and increasing life expectancy. However, many of these new advances included potent pharmaceuticals and highly invasive surgical procedures (open-heart surgery, brain surgery, etc.) which carry increased risk of complications. Many of these complications are serious or even life-threatening. Then, as now, when things turn out badly, it is human nature to look for someone to blame.

On the legal front, the growing use of medical malpractice insurance by physicians made taking on medical negligence cases a potentially profitable activity for lawyers. This is not to criticize ethical attorneys taking on a case of legitimate medical malpractice for a client. However, there was evidence of widespread abuse with frivolous malpractice suits being filed. There were cases in the early days of the malpractice crisis in which a lawyer would file a lawsuit or simply write a letter threatening to sue, and the doctor's insurance company would settle these "nuisance cases" out of court for a relatively

---

30   Bal, Sonny G. "An Introduction to Medical Malpractice in the United States." Clinical Orthopaedics and Related Research 467, no. 2 (November 26, 2008): 339-47. https://doi.org/10.1007/s11999-008-0636-2.

small amount. This was a business decision based on the fact that this expense was less than the cost of taking a clearly winnable case to court. The physician might have had no say in this decision or simply agreed in order to avoid months or years of aggravation. Fortunately, insurance companies and physicians began to understand that settling nuisance cases out of court merely encouraged more of the same, and this practice is no longer common.

In the decades after the 1960s, there were a series of extremely large jury awards in the multimillion-dollar range. In addition, there was an overall increase in the number of lawsuits filed, both legitimate and those without merit. This created a rapid rise in the rate of medical malpractice insurance premiums. Surgeons and obstetricians were particularly affected by this, and as a result, many made the decision to no longer practice medicine. Other physicians decided to not carry insurance.

These circumstances prompted over 30 state legislatures to enact legal measures known as "tort reform" to deal with what was widely considered a crisis. These reforms are complex and vary greatly from state to state. Among the most common reforms is a financial limit on "non-economic damages," which includes pain and suffering. These measures are controversial, and some lawyers and consumer advocates argue that it is unfair to individuals of legitimate malpractice. However, in those states, such as Texas, with the most robust reforms, there is evidence that these measures are easing the crisis by lowering the cost of malpractice insurance premiums paid by physicians and fewer lawsuits being filed.[31]

Reforms and controversies aside, there is no question that medical malpractice creates a loss of vital trust in the doc-

---

31   Berlin, Joey. "Coming of Age: Celebrating 15 Years of Texas Tort Reform." Texas Medicine. Last modified September 14, 2018. https://doi.org/10.1007/s11999-008-0636-2.

tor-patient relationship by both parties. It would be desirable for all involved if malpractice could be eliminated altogether. However, this is unrealistic as healthcare providers can never be expected to be perfect or completely free from errors in judgment. The best solution would be a fair and balanced system in which an individual harmed due to a negligent decision by a physician could receive just compensation, and a physician could be assured that he or she would be immune from legal action for a bad outcome when the standard of care is shown to have been met.

Until, and if, this idealized system becomes reality, there are important proactive steps for the healthcare consumer to take in assessing a choice of healthcare providers. These include:

- Obtaining knowledge of any excessive malpractice activity in a physician's history. As referenced in chapter 3, an internet background check through your state board of medical examiners provides malpractice history for physicians in most cases.
- Asking for an explanation of any recommended tests or procedures that seem excessive to you.
- Requesting a second opinion if there is any doubt or concern in your mind.

CHAPTER 8

Poor Communication

"The single biggest problem in communication is the illusion that it has taken place."
—George Bernard Shaw

"We were given two ears and one mouth so that we can listen twice as much as we speak."
—Epictetus (Greek philosopher)

These two quotes speak to the ancient and universal problem with human communication. However, communication is the lifeblood of the doctor-patient relationship and should never be an illusion. The idealized version of doctor-patient communication was briefly discussed previously in chapter 3 under the topic of bedside manner. Numerous scientific studies have shown that outcomes of medical treatment are directly impacted by the quality of communication between doctor and patient. This goes directly to the matter of trust and satisfaction for both the patient and the physician. This chapter deals in detail with each of the following specific issues related to doctor-patient communication that may adversely affect levels of trust and satisfaction in the relationship:

- Inequality in listening and speaking
- Failing to speak in understandable terms—"medical language" vs "everyday language"
- Inadequate translation resources when there is not a shared native language
- Failure to accommodate speech, hearing, or sight impediments
- Not accounting for a patient's literacy levels
- Poor nonverbal communication
- Failure to communicate between providers.

The potential for inequality in the doctor-patient relationship has been mentioned earlier. This is never desirable but is especially problematic in the critical area of communication. In a typical doctor-patient encounter, it is common for the physician to open the conversation. Ideally this should involve an initial exchange of pleasantries, after which the physician inquires what the patient would like to discuss. Then what should follow is a free-flowing back-and-forth exchange characterized by concentrated and respectful listening and careful choice of language and tone. However, this is not always the case. A number of research studies have discovered that it takes the average physician less than 30 seconds to interrupt and redirect a patient's conversation.[32] There are some circumstances in which it is appropriate for the doctor to "guide" the conversation with the purpose of leading to a correct diagnosis, but early, abrupt, or frequent

---

32 Phillips, Kari A., and Naykky, S. Ospina. "Physicians Interrupting Patients." Journal of the American Medical Association 318, no. 1 (July 2017): 93-94. https://doi.org/doi:10.1001/jama.2017.6493.

interruption is clearly counterproductive to a high-quality healthcare encounter.

Another communication problem is the physician speaking in "medical language" versus common everyday language. Terms such as *myocardial infarction, onychomycosis,* and *atelectasis* are common knowledge for physicians, but this type of medical jargon can be very confusing to most laypersons. Doctors are immersed in this medical language for years in their training before entering medical practice and continue to use it with colleagues for a lifetime. It therefore takes a conscious effort not to slip into using medical language with patients.

It is the responsibility of the doctor to translate medical language into lay language. Patients should always ask for a translation if needed, but many may feel shy or embarrassed to do so. However, the bottom line is that healthcare delivery and outcomes are compromised if a patient does not comprehend a doctor's explanation of a condition or its recommended treatment.

In our multicultural society, there is also the common occurrence of the doctor and patient not having a shared native, or first, language. If the physician is not fluent in the patient's preferred language, adequate translation resources from family, staff, or advocates must be available. Related to this issue is the need to accommodate any impediments in hearing, speech, or sight. It goes without saying that if a patient cannot comprehend the doctor's words, there is no possibility of achieving the desired outcome. In fact, there is a strong probability of misinterpretation and great potential for harm.

Another sensitive communication issue relates to patient literacy levels. Literacy goes well beyond the ability to read and write. The United Nations Educational, Scientific and Cultural Organization (UNESCO) defines basic general *literacy* as the "ability to identify, understand, interpret, create, communicate and compute, using printed and written materials associated with varying contexts." *The current gov-*

ernment (health.gov) definition of health literacy is "the degree to which individuals have the capacity to obtain, process, and understand basic *health* information and services needed to make appropriate *health* decisions." The following summary and statistics from a national survey are disturbing:[33]

- Four levels of literacy were assessed: proficient (best), intermediate, basic, and below basic (worst).
- Only 12% of adults were found to be functioning at a proficient (best) health literacy level.
- The level of education made a difference, but still only 30% of those with a bachelor's degree were found to be proficient (best).
- A staggering 77 million adult Americans tested as basic or below basic literacy levels.

A commonly overlooked communication issue involves nonverbal communication. Experts have concluded that appropriate nonverbal communication is extremely important in promoting understanding and that poor nonverbal communication can have a negative effect. Nonverbal communication includes physical appearance, eye contact, posture, gestures, facial expression, tone of voice, and touch. The best way to illustrate the importance of nonverbal communication is to draw a comparison. Consider the outcome of a health encounter with a physician who engages a patient with neat and appropriate attire, good eye contact (not staring down), upright posture, a calm tone of voice, pleasant facial expression and, if appropriate, placing a reassuring hand on the shoulder. Compare this to the effect of a physician who

---

33 "America's Health Literacy: Why We Need Accessible Health Information." U.S. Department of Health and Human Services. Last modified 2008. https://health.gov/communication/literacy/issuebrief/.

is disheveled in appearance, avoids eye contact, slumps over, appears rushed and indifferent, speaks harshly or arrogantly, and avoids any physical contact including a handshake. It is fortunately rare to confront this latter example, but a patient should immediately switch physicians if it ever does occur.

There is a final potential communication problem that does not occur directly between doctor and patient but is nevertheless critically important in healthcare delivery. This involves communication among different healthcare providers caring for the same patient. This may be demonstrated by the following common scenario involving a patient with a complex medical problem:

A patient is seen by a family physician, who decides to refer the patient to a specialist for further evaluation. This specialist then determines the patient needs to be admitted to the hospital, where the care is overseen by a different specialist known as a hospitalist. There are often other specialists involved in a hospital stay as well. The patient may then be transferred to a rehabilitation facility under the care of yet another physician. When discharged from the rehab facility, the patient must then follow up with the primary care provider.

In a perfect healthcare world, all the physicians involved in such a scenario will have communicated and made their findings and records available to one another.

This is what is termed "continuity of care," and it is not uncommon for there to be gaps in this process. It is estimated that poor continuity of care is the source of many medical errors and the basis for as much as 30 percent of malpractice cases.[34] The only way a patient (or person advocating for a

---

34 Schleiter, Kristin E. "Difficult Patient-Physician Relationships and the Risk of Medical Malpractice Litigation." AMA Journal of Ethics. https://doi.org/10.1001/virtualmentor.2009.11.3.hlaw1-0903.

patient when the patient is not able) can be certain if this continuity of care is being carried out is to be aware of the issue and request evidence that every provider and facility involved in caregiving is communicating properly.

There are no internet resources that can alert a healthcare consumer to any of the above communication problems in a healthcare provider. Patient awareness of the signs of poor communication is crucial, and it is worth repeating that list of warning signs here:

- Inequality in listening and speaking
- Failing to speak in understandable terms— "medical language" vs "everyday language"
- Inadequate translation resources when there is not a shared native language
- Failure to accommodate speech, hearing, or sight impediments
- Not accounting for patient literacy levels
- Poor nonverbal communication
- Failure to communicate between providers.

If one or more of these problems are identified and cannot be corrected through direct communication and negotiation with the healthcare provider, it is cause to change providers.

CHAPTER 9

Physician Arrogance

Our society has chosen to confer considerable respect and esteem upon physicians, most of whom do not abuse this high privilege. However, some physicians become arrogant. Arrogance is an unflattering personality trait that is characterized by self-importance, conceit, and egotism. It often manifests as impatience and frustration and reflects an attitude of superiority. Ironically, psychologists believe arrogance to be caused at least in part by a sense of personal insecurity and fear that others will actually see flaws or weaknesses if a false front of superiority is not maintained. Whatever the causes, professional and personal arrogance in a physician does not contribute to trustworthiness as a healthcare provider. To the contrary, it can lead to harm in several ways discussed below.

At the other end of the personality spectrum from arrogance is the very desirable trait of humility. Humility is often incorrectly perceived to be weakness. In fact, the word is derived from "humus," which is Latin for "earth." Therefore, a more appropriate description of a humble person is "down to earth" or "well grounded." This is precisely the type of personality trait that is associated with trustworthiness.

It is important to distinguish between confidence and arrogance. Patients need to feel confident in the recommendations from their physician, and the physician needs to have confidence in his or her professional knowledge and skill. If a given physician projects confidence in making healthcare recommendations and simultaneously displays humility, the patient is likely to feel reassured. If another physician offers the same recommendations, but projects arrogance, the patient may feel humiliated and demeaned. This is counterproductive to achieving the gold standard in the doctor-patient relationship, which is a partnership with shared decision-making.

Since arrogance involves a sense of superiority and a tendency to become frustrated and impatient with others, patients may unknowingly enable an arrogance-prone physician. Placing such a doctor on a pedestal or being passive in the relationship can encourage the stereotypical doctor "God complex," which is the ultimate in arrogance. Also, physicians can become frustrated with patients who disregard sound medical advice and follow unproven, potentially dangerous advice from a family member or magazine article. A non-arrogant physician will not allow these common actions to provoke an obvious display of frustration or condescending attitude, whereas such behavior will serve as fuel for an arrogant healthcare provider. This is just another good reason for patients not to be passive or submissive, but to instead establish a partnership with their doctor.

There are also factors in medical education that may contribute to physician arrogance. Although there have been improvements in recent years, physicians in training can be treated as virtual indentured servants with long hours and low pay. It is also not rare for providers in training to be under the supervision of arrogant individuals. As a result, some physicians emerge from this experience having taken on the arrogant and abusive behavior to which they were subjected.

Computerized medical records are a technological advance in healthcare delivery that has some significant benefits. However, if a physician is entering data into a laptop or PC during a healthcare encounter, rather than maintaining eye contact, the physician's physical focus on the electronic device can convey a message to the patient of indifference and lack of concern. Also, physicians are contending with more governmental regulations and bureaucratic red tape than ever before. This can create a sense of being rushed and distracted, which may translate as arrogance to a patient who understandably is expecting undivided attention.

The greatest risk for harm from physician arrogance involves interaction with other healthcare providers. A small number of arrogant doctors exhibit verbal, and even physical, abuse toward colleagues. This is typically directed at a colleague or coworker in a subordinate position. An example would be an arrogant senior surgeon verbally abusing a surgical resident in training for questioning a decision. A more common example occurs when a nurse questions an arrogant doctor's action. There are documented cases of physicians throwing surgical instruments in the operating suite or charts in a nursing station.

These activities are clearly workplace violence and are the equivalent of road rage. When such activities go unchecked, it can create an atmosphere of fear and intimidation for the subordinate healthcare professionals involved. This can lead to situations where an arrogant physician's mistakes are recognized by subordinate healthcare workers, but not reported in order to avoid abusive behavior. This unquestionably contributes to preventable medical errors.

Although this abusive activity still occurs, it is much less frequent due to a zero-tolerance policy for this behavior in most healthcare facilities. There are systems in place to report abusive behavior. If the investigation confirms a problem, the physician is generally required to seek professional help and is placed on probation and peer review until there is evidence that there has been a change in behavior. If the behavior involves physical assault, criminal charges are possible, and the person's medical license may be suspended or revoked.

Recognizing an arrogant physician is usually not difficult for a patient. Of course, anyone can have a bad day, and it would not be fair to judge a person based on a brief encounter. However, considering the potential dangers described above, any clear pattern of impatience, indifference, condescension, or other characteristics of arrogance is cause to consider looking for another doctor.

CHAPTER 10

Role of the Patient in the Relationship of Trust

The previous chapters have focused primarily on characteristics of healthcare providers which are necessary to produce trustworthiness and contribute to the development of a high-quality doctor-patient relationship. Ideally this relationship will exist as a shared decision-making partnership. Therefore, it is also important to discuss the responsibilities of the patient that are required in order to complete this ideal relationship.

First among these important responsibilities is not being passive in the doctor-patient relationship. The best outcomes of medical treatment result from shared decision-making and require an engaged and proactive patient. While it is important to have confidence in the advice of the physician, it is also important for a patient to feel free to ask questions, offer suggestions, and ultimately make the final decision in all healthcare matters.

There are many things that affect a person's ability or willingness to be engaged and active in a healthcare encounter. Individual personality type is a significant factor. Some patients are naturally outgoing and communicative, while others are naturally reserved or shy. The reason for the healthcare encounter also plays a major role. It is easier to be active and engaged when the reason is minor, such as a routine physical or an uncomplicated sore throat. However, it can become quite difficult if the encounter is for a serious symptom or sensitive matter, such as chest pain or sexual dysfunction. Some of the issues discussed in the chapter on communication, such as health literacy and physical impediments (hearing, speech, sight), can impact the level of patient engagement in an encounter as well.

Regardless of the basic personal characteristics or the reason for the healthcare encounter, there are certain methods that can improve the interaction with the physician and achieve the desired goal of shared decision-making. A patient should approach a healthcare encounter with two major goals:

- Provide the physician with a clear understanding of the reason for the visit
- Leave the encounter with a detailed and clear understanding of shared decisions and medical recommendations.

The most effective way to achieve these goals is to make notes before, during, and after the encounter.

There is a proverb that states that "the shortest pencil is better than the longest memory." This correctly conveys the fact that writing down information is superior to human memory. This is particularly true when the information that needs to be recalled is complex or the situation in which the information is obtained is stressful as is often the case in a healthcare encounter.

It is a good idea to prepare for an upcoming office visit by making a list of concerns or questions you want to cover during the encounter. You should present this list to your provider early in the visit and together determine an approach to address the questions or concerns based on priority. If the list is long, it may be necessary to schedule an additional appointment. Before the encounter ends, you should check off those issues that have been fully covered or resolved and keep the remainder for future reference. You should also write down notes about the answers and recommendations your provider gives. You should review these notes later and note any additional questions that may need to be addressed in future encounters.

Even if you, the patient, depart with a written summary of the encounter, it is a very good idea to verbally express this information back to the provider. Along these lines, there is a current effort in medical education to promote the routine incorporation of a technique known as "teach-back" at the end of each encounter.[35] This involves the provider summarizing the recommendations and instructions and then asking patients to repeat them back in their own words. This can be supplemented by printed reference or instructional material for patients to take home. When all these written and verbal safeguards are incorporated into a doctor-patient encounter, it markedly reduces both the chance of misunderstanding and the potential for medical errors and bad outcomes.

Another effective way to enhance the level of communication and understanding in a healthcare encounter is to take a trusted family member or friend with you as a personal advocate. This is particularly valuable if the problems to be addressed involve serious, stressful, or emotional issues. It is

---

[35] "Health Literacy Universal Precautions Toolkit, 2nd; Use the Teach-Back Method: Tool #5 Edition." U.S. Department of Health and Human Services. Last modified February 2015. https://www.ahrq.gov/health-literacy/quality-resources/tools/literacy-toolkit/healthlittoolkit2-tool5.html.

also especially helpful to have an advocate present if there are hearing, vision, speech, or first-language impediments.

When physician recommendations include complex, invasive, or expensive tests or procedures, it is entirely appropriate for a patient to request a second or third opinion. Some patients may be reluctant to ask for this out of concern for offending the physician, but this should not be a concern. If the first physician consulted is offended by the request for an additional opinion, this should serve as a red flag to the patient. Any trustworthy physician will not take offense and will instead encourage additional professional input. This is in the best interest of both the patient and the physician and will increase the probability of the best outcome possible.

There is another somewhat sensitive issue for patients to consider when their physician recommends expensive testing or procedures. This involves having the physician fully disclose any ownership he or she may have in the facility performing the test or procedure. There may be legitimate reasons for a physician to have a financial interest in such a facility. He or she may believe that the quality of the testing or safety of the procedure is superior and is therefore beneficial for patients.

However, there are statistics that indicate self-referrals may result in unnecessary testing. The Government Accounting Office (GAO) conducted a review of this subject from 2004-2010. It studied the referral patterns to MRI, CT scans, pathology labs (for biopsies), and radiation treatment facilities. The findings revealed substantial increases in referrals to these facilities from physicians who had a financial interest compared to physicians who did not. The conclusion of the study was: "Financial incentives for self-referring providers were likely a major factor driving the increase in referrals."[36]

---

36 "Higher Use of Advanced Imaging Services by Providers Who Self-Refer Costing Medicare Millions." United States

There have been laws on the books for years that either restrict physician ownership in facilities to which they refer patients or require full disclosure of their financial interest to patients. However, there are also many "exceptions" (some would say loopholes) to these laws that make it difficult to prevent abuse. It is very hard for patients to be fully aware when they are the subjects of these self-referrals.

The best approach for a patient in dealing with this issue is to address this with the physician *before* it ever arises. If a patient or family member waits until the time of a referral for a test or procedure, the circumstances at that point may be so stressful or emotional that the tendency is to proceed without questioning. Ideally, this issue should be covered in the initial process of selecting a physician as part of the background check that was discussed in a previous chapter. However, it is never too late to ask for this information. An ethical physician will gladly disclose the reasons why he or she has a financial interest in the facility to which the self-referral has been made, and the patient can then decide whether to proceed or not. If the physician takes offense when asked for the disclosure, it should raise the same red flag as objecting to a second opinion.

The American Medical Association has developed the following written policy on patient rights and responsibilities, and it is worth reviewing here:[37]

Government Accountability Office. Last modified September, 2012. https://www.gao.gov/assets/650/648988.pdf.

37 "AMA Code of Medical Ethics Opinions on Patient-Physician Relationships." JAMA. https://www.ama-assn.org/sites/ama-assn.org/files/corp/media-browser/code-of-medical-ethics-chapter-1.pdf.

Code of Medical Ethics Opinion 1.1.4

Successful medical care requires ongoing collaboration between patients and physicians. Their partnership requires both individuals to take an active role in the healing process.

Independent, competent patients control the decisions that direct their health care. With that exercise of self-governance and choice comes several responsibilities. Patients contribute to the collaborative effort when they:

(a) Are truthful and forthcoming with their physicians and strive to express their concerns clearly. Physicians likewise should encourage patients to raise questions or concerns.

(b) Provide as complete a medical history as they can, including providing information about past illnesses, medications, hospitalizations, family history of illness, and other matters relating to present health.

(c) Cooperate with agreed-on treatment plans. Since adhering to treatment is often essential to public and individual safety, patients should disclose whether they have or have not followed the agreed-on plan and indicate when they would like to reconsider the plan.

(d) Accept care from medical students, residents, and other trainees under appropriate supervision. Participation in medical education is to the mutual benefit of patients and the healthcare system; nonetheless, patients' refusal of care by a trainee should be respected in keeping with ethics guidance.

(e) Meet their financial responsibilities with regard to medical care or discuss financial hardships with their physicians. Patients should be aware of costs associated with using a limited resource like health care and try to use medical resources carefully.

(f) Recognize that a healthy lifestyle can often prevent or lessen illness and take responsibility to follow preventive measures and adopt health-enhancing behaviors.
(g) Be aware of and refrain from behavior that unreasonably places the health of others at risk. They should ask about what they can do to prevent transmission of infectious disease.
(h) Refrain from being disruptive in the clinical setting.
(i) Not knowingly initiate or participate in medical fraud.
(j) Report illegal or unethical behavior by physicians or other healthcare professionals to the appropriate medical societies, licensing boards, or law enforcement authorities.

This chapter concludes the section that addresses the first two major goals of this book as stated in chapter 1:

- *Explaining in detail the scope of the trust problem*
- *Providing the reader with information that may be used to evaluate a healthcare provider for trustworthiness.*

The following six chapters will focus on the third major goal:

- *Helping the average healthcare consumer have a better understanding of medical economics.*

CHAPTER 11

Will Americans Be Able to Afford Health Care in the 21ˢᵗ Century?

In spite of a recent slowing trend, the cost of health care in the United States has been growing at a rate greater than inflation for decades. Spending for medical services now comprises about 17.8 percent of the gross domestic product (the total value of everything produced in the country). This has dramatically increased from 5 percent in 1960. The actual dollar amount has increased at an even greater rate to $11,500 per person, compared to $146 per person in 1960.[38]

---

38 "National Health Expenditure Data." Centers for Medicare and Medicaid Services. Last modified December 17, 2019. https://www.cms.gov/Research-Statistics-Data-and-Systems/Statistics-Trends-and-Reports/NationalHealthExpendData/NationalHealthAccountsHistorical.

The U.S. spends far more on health care than any other industrialized nation. A recent Texas Medical Association poll revealed how significantly these rising costs affect individuals and their ability to access needed health care:[39]

- 55% of Texans say it's difficult for them to pay for health care, including more than 27% who say it's "very difficult"
- 60% say that someone in their household skipped or postponed healthcare needs in the past 12 months
- 33% skipped a recommended test or treatment
- 31% didn't fill a prescription
- 22% cut pills in half or skipped doses
- 15% had problems getting mental health care.

There is virtually universal agreement that these rising costs cannot be sustained without having serious adverse effects on the health of individuals and bankrupting this nation in the process. The solution to this problem has been debated for decades. The fact that there has not been any sustained progress speaks to the complexity of medical economics in the United States.

Our experience and observations as practicing family practitioners over almost five decades indicate that neither the average healthcare consumer nor the average politician dealing with healthcare legislation and regulations have a clear understanding of the root causes of the disproportionate rise in costs. This is all complicated by the current heightened political polarization. Until this situation changes, there can be no meaningful reforms effected. Fortunately, even in this unsettled environment, it is possible for an informed and pro-

---

39 Amadeo, Kimberly. "The Rising Cost of Health Care by Year and Its Causes." The Balance. Last modified January 14, 2020. https://www.thebalance.com/causes-of-rising-health care-costs-4064878.

active healthcare consumer to avoid being overwhelmed with medical expenses.

If you are an average employed U.S. citizen, you should be able to afford the health care necessary throughout your life span **if** the following conditions are met:

- You understand that there will be predictable costs for your basic healthcare needs and possible additional expenses for unforeseen medical events such as a major emergency or chronic illness
- You wisely budget and plan for these expenses just as you would do for shelter, food, transportation, etc.
- You know when (and when NOT) to access the healthcare system
- When you do decide to access the healthcare system, you make the correct choice of provider and facility
- You understand how to determine if any healthcare recommendation you receive is based on scientific evidence and is truly necessary, thereby avoiding inappropriate medical testing and treatment
- You make lifestyle choices that maximize your chances for good health and longevity and avoid those choices that have the opposite effect
- You understand that the medical economics system in the U.S. does not always follow basic free market economic principles and you use that knowledge to adjust your decisions as a healthcare consumer accordingly.

The next few chapters will seek to clarify and simplify the major causes of the current healthcare cost crisis. This will include some proposed solutions to deal with these causes and assist all individuals in obtaining affordable, high-quality care throughout their life span without waiting for political solutions that may be years away.

CHAPTER 12

What Is Causing the High Cost of Health Care?

The solution to almost any problem requires a clear understanding of the cause or causes of that problem. There are many reasons behind the very high cost of health care in this country, and it is beyond the scope of this book to cover all of them in detail. However, we will discuss the following major factors that are driving many of the high costs:

- An aging population
- An increase in the prevalence of chronic diseases
- A severe shortage of doctors
- A decrease of people in the workforce paying taxes
- Lack of adequate "consumerism" in health care
- Overuse of medical resources with questionable value, especially some expensive high-tech imaging and surgical procedures

- Underuse of less costly medical resources with proven effectiveness, especially preventive care and humane end-of-life care.

The law of supply and demand in a free market generally dictates that the cost of a product or service will rise in the face of an increase in demand or a decrease in supply. The remainder of this chapter will address the first four causes of high healthcare costs. Two of these causes involve *supply* problems (a physician shortage and too few persons in the workforce) and two involve *demand* problems (an aging population and the chronic disease epidemic). These four factors combine to provide the basis for a perfect storm for higher healthcare costs.

The statistics regarding the aging of the U.S. population and the accompanying increase in demand for healthcare services are staggering, as indicated by the following:[40]

- There are currently 54 million Americans over the age of 65, which is 16% of the total population, compared to 9.5% in 1966.
- This number will increase to 75 million (21% of the population) by 2030, as the remainder of 79 million baby boomers turn 65.
- In addition to the increased number of people entering their senior years, seniors are living longer, with an increase in life expectancy of five years since 1970.

---

40 "Texans' Experiences with Affordability of and Access to Health Care." Episcopal Health Foundation. Last modified June 2019. https://www.episcopalhealth.org/files/3815/6044/2653/Texans_Experiences_with_Health_Care_Affordability_and_Access_2019_FINALjune.pdf.

- With increased age comes an increased rate of chronic health conditions, and these conditions consume 85% of healthcare spending (it should be stated here that an increase in the prevalence of chronic disease is not limited to seniors but is occurring in all age groups, including children).
- Less than 10% of persons entering Medicare at age 65 have multiple (more than five) chronic diseases, but by age 85, this percentage increases to 25%.

This increased demand for health care would be bad enough on its own, but there are additional problems on the supply side of the equation as these facts indicate:[41]

- At the same time that the population is aging, there is a decrease in the birth rate and net population growth in the U.S.
- By the year 2035, it is projected that for the first time in our history there will be more persons over age 65 than persons under age 18.
- When Medicare came into existence in 1965 there were 4.6 workers for every retiree; with current trends, this will drop to half that level by 2030.
- This reversal in the young-to-old ratio creates a major problem for financing Medicare because the taxes paid by workers that go to help sustain this type of government program decrease in the face of the increased demand on the program.

Another serious problem on the supply side of healthcare services is the estimate that there will be a shortage of

---

41 Doherty, Tucker. "Medicare's time bomb, in 7 charts." Politico, September 12, 2018. https://www.politico.com/agenda/story/2018/09/12/medicare-baby-boomers-trust-fund-000694.

90,000 doctors by 2025.[42] Among the reasons for this is the fact that there has not been enough of an increase in medical residency programs to train new physicians to meet the increased demand, particularly in primary care. This is worsened by the increasing trend of many currently practicing physicians leaving the profession early as a result of burnout due to stress and professional dissatisfaction.

Some of these individuals remain in the medical field but move into administrative roles or other areas of non-patient care. Others change professions entirely or take early retirement. In any case, the net effect is to add to the shortage of physicians providing direct patient care. These are the results of a recent survey of physicians in Texas that mirror similar national survey results:[43]

- 61.2% said their morale and feelings about the current state of the medical profession were somewhat or very negative
- 69.1% said they were somewhat or very negative/pessimistic about the future of the profession
- 52% said they would not recommend medicine as a career to their children or other young people
- 54.5% said they plan to accelerate their retirement because of changes in health care

---

42   Berlin, Joey. "Battling Burnout." Texas Medical Association. Last modified April 2018. https://www.texmed.org/BattlingBurnout/.
43   Kamal, Rabah, Daniel McDermott, and Cynthia Cox. "How has U.S. Spending on Healthcare Changed Over Time?" Health System Tracker. Last modified December 20, 2019. https://www.healthsystemtracker.org/chart-collection/u-s-spending-health care-changed-time/#item-nhe-trends_per-capita-out-of-pocket-expenditures-1970-2018.

- The top answers when asked for the two least satisfying factors affecting professional satisfaction:

    — Regulatory/paperwork burdens (64.1%)
    — Having medical decisions controlled by insurance company policy or government regulations (36.5%).

Even though these supply and demand problems paint a bleak picture, there are some practical solutions to some of the above issues. These solutions are not easy and will require major commitments on both the individual and societal level. These solutions will be addressed in the final chapter of the book, along with solutions to the problem areas dealt with in the next three chapters.

CHAPTER 13

The Lack of Consumerism in Health Care

For the purposes of this book, this is the definition we will be using for the term *consumerism*:

> *a modern movement to promote the maximum involvement of the consumer in making purchases for goods and services, and to protect the consumer against useless, inferior, or dangerous products, misleading advertising, unfair pricing, etc.*[44]

This movement has been present in most segments of the U.S. economy for decades but has only recently become somewhat active in health care. However, consumerism in

---

44   Consumerism. (2020). In: Dictionary.com. [online] Available at: https://www.dictionary.com/browse/consumerism?s=t [Accessed 6 Feb. 2020].

the area of medical services still lags far behind its presence in the general market economy. The following information is intended to define how pervasive "anti-consumerism" is in the area of medical economics.

There are reasonable explanations for some of the lack of consumerism in healthcare purchases. Our bodies are much more complex, mysterious, and unpredictable than our cars, houses, etc. There is also the emotional component involving our health that is absent with most other consumer items. We rightfully place a higher value on our health versus the value of regular consumer goods. If our car is totaled in an accident or our house is badly damaged, we probably shop around for qualified persons or facilities to do the needed work. We are much less likely to shop around when there is an equivalent issue with our health, such as a bad injury or suspected heart problem. Nevertheless, there are many aspects of health care in which we could, and should, apply the same basic consumer skills we use for other purchases.

To better illustrate this, it may prove useful to describe how consumers deal with most purchases and compare this to healthcare purchases. When we need food, we go to the grocery store and pay with cash or a credit card. The same process applies to clothing, entertainment, etc. For large purchases, we may take out an automobile loan or home mortgage. However, in all these instances, consumers pay for these goods and services with out-of-pocket money. For wise consumers, this requires careful decisions as to what they need or want to purchase. These decisions are ideally made by comparison shopping and using a wide variety of resources available to assess the quality and reliability of a potential purchase, as well as the integrity of the individual or company providing the product or service. These resources create the transparency that is critical to making informed decisions as a consumer. In addition, effective consumerism involves a household budget plan that guides purchases based on what the level of a given household income will support.

Imagine buying any product or service without full knowledge in advance of the cost or quality and then basically having no easy recourse for a refund if the product or service proves ineffective. Then add to this a lack of choice about where you can purchase the product or service. Most American consumers would not tolerate these conditions. However, this is what occurs on a regular basis for a large percentage of our population when paying for healthcare services.

The amount of healthcare expenses that are paid for with out-of-pocket money is currently just over 10 percent. Although rising somewhat in recent years, the historic trend is that this percentage has fallen significantly over time.[45] This is not meant to imply that the average American does not pay for his or her health care. We do ultimately pay one way or the other, but unlike with food, clothing, etc., we are often not aware of how this happens. This is primarily because much of the money spent on health care is tied to a private or governmental health "insurance" policy. The word insurance is in quotation marks because health insurance arguably is not truly insurance.

We will use this definition of traditional insurance taken from several dictionary and insurance industry sources:

> *a policy that ensures full or partial financial compensation for loss or damage **beyond the control** of the insured party in exchange for a premium.*

---

45   "Health Savings Accounts and Other Tax-Favored Health Plans." Department of the Treasury. Last modified 2018. https://www.irs.gov/pub/irs-pdf/p969.pdf.

This definition fits an auto, home, or life insurance policy. These forms of traditional insurance do not compensate people for damages that have already occurred and typically cover only unpredictable and unexpected damages or events. They generally do not cover things considered to be routine maintenance. In addition, there will be an increase in an insurance premium if the risk for the insured entity (auto, home, life) is above average. In some cases, a traditional policy cannot be obtained at all if the insurance company judges the risk to be too great.

For instance, one cannot purchase an automobile insurance policy and expect payment to repair damages from an accident that occurred prior to the date the policy went into effect (a "preexisting condition" in the vehicle). Also, no one expects their auto insurance to pay for tune-ups or to replace worn-out tires. There is no expectation that homeowners insurance will pay for fertilizing the yard or cover the cost of repainting the exterior. Everyone understands that life insurance premiums will be higher (or unavailable) if the insured engages in high-risk behavior such as smoking or sky-diving and people are generally aware that auto insurance rates will be higher if a person has had multiple accidents. Traditional policies for life, home, and auto are "owned" by the insured and are "portable." This means the policy stays in effect as long as the premiums are paid regardless of a change in address, job, or family situation.

The above definition and description of traditional insurance fits only a fraction of the typical health insurance policies written today. The one area in which a healthcare policy *does* meet the definition of traditional insurance is in its payment of covered medical expenses for an accident or unforeseen illness. It differs from traditional insurance in most all the other characteristics in the previous paragraphs:

- It does cover conditions that are not beyond the control of the insured

- It does cover maintenance (expected) conditions
- It does cover preexisting conditions
- It has no dollar limit on coverage
- Most policies are not portable.

Under current federal law, health insurance must not exclude preexisting conditions and there is no lifetime limit allowed on the amount of coverage. Just imagine what would happen to insurance rates for automobiles or homes if those policies were required to pay for maintenance expenses or the repair of damages incurred by an auto or home before the policy went into effect, and there was no dollar limit to the amount of coverage. Those costs would have to be passed on to the insured individuals through increased premiums. This is exactly what has occurred with health insurance and explains much of the increase in these health policy premiums.

Also, most health policies now will reimburse for a rather long list of *expected*, or maintenance, health expenses, such as annual physicals and vaccinations. This has the well-meaning intention of encouraging people to avail themselves of preventive medical care. However, since these are expected and/or maintenance expenses, this portion of a health insurance policy is much more of a "prepaid income subsidy" than true insurance. It would seem to be much more efficient to allow the money devoted to these expenses to remain in the pockets of the insured individuals, thereby avoiding the waste of the extra administrative costs (estimated to be as high as 30 percent) that are inevitable in this arrangement. Reforming these aspects of health insurance would then permit the healthcare policy both to cost less for the insured and to fulfill its true role as insurance by covering unexpected events such as an accident or serious illness.

There have been some attempts to deal with this issue in the healthcare insurance field, such as "health savings accounts" (HSAs), flexible savings accounts (FSAs), and health reimbursement arrangements (HRAs).[46] These arrangements accomplish some of the desired goal of having the consumer pay for services more directly, but they are not universally available in health insurance policies.

Another anti-consumerism element of many health insurance policies is the lack of choice in how to use the coverage for which most individuals pay a large monthly health insurance premium, either through their employer or to the federal government in the case of Medicare. Although there are some health insurance policies that permit complete freedom of choice of healthcare provider and/or facility, many policies come with some restrictions on the choice of where and from whom the insured individual receives health care.

With these particular policies, there is a requirement that you pick from a healthcare provider that is in the insurance network. If you go outside of this network, you may not be covered or must pay a much greater price for the service. In addition, when it becomes necessary to obtain healthcare services beyond the doctor's office visit (hospital, emergency room, lab, imaging, etc.), the insurance company often has the final say as to whether the recommended service is covered. If it is covered, there is frequently no choice as to which facility provides the service, as the facility must also be "in network."

Finally, there is the serious problem of the lack of "portability" with many health insurance policies. Portability allows an insurance policy to remain in effect as long as premiums are paid and is not affected by a change in employment, marital status, or address. This occurs primarily with policies provided by employers for their employees, and it includes the largest percentage of Americans with health insurance.

---

46 Evans, Robert G. "Waste, Economists and American Healthcare." Healthcare Policy 9, no. 2 (November 2013): 12-20. https://www.ncbi.nlm.nih.gov/pmc/articles/PMC3999538/.

The tradition of employers providing health insurance for employees goes back many decades, when employers were attempting to attract workers and avoid the wage and price controls following World War II by offering the benefit of health coverage. Since that time, the tax laws have been written to encourage this arrangement. In the mid-twentieth century, when health care was much less expensive and many people worked for the same employer until retirement, this seemed to work for the most part. However, today we are faced with skyrocketing healthcare costs and a work force in which people change jobs on a very frequent basis.

Unlike with auto, life, or home insurance, in many cases an individual must change health insurance coverage whenever he or she changes employer. Also, if a married couple has insurance with one of their employers and divorce or death occurs, one person must change health insurance. There have been some attempts to lessen this issue with the HIPAA law[47] and the Affordable Care Act (Obamacare)[48], but these portability provisions are more of a temporary fix than a real solution. Many of the current legislative healthcare reform proposals attempt to correct this problem, but the current political climate does not create much optimism that consensus can be reached on this or many of the other pressing problems in the complex world of medical economics. This makes it doubly important for each individual to become informed and able to take advantage of the best available options that are currently available.

Another anti-consumerism characteristic in health care is not knowing the costs of many services before they are

---

47 HIPPA portability: https://www.phpni.com/policies/portability#:~:text=The%20HIPAA%20portability%20provision%2C%20as,iss...
https://www.phpni.com/policies/portability
48 ACA portability: https://www.nfib.com/cribsheets/portability/

obtained. Ask yourself if you were aware in advance of the **true** cost (not just your co-pay) of your last doctor's office visit. Not only is this information commonly a mystery for this most basic of healthcare encounters, but that mystery is multiplied many times over for an emergency room encounter or a hospital stay.

Ironically, it can be even more confusing to understand the cost of services even after they have been obtained. If you need proof, just look at your most recent explanation of benefits from your insurance company, sent to you after the encounter. Worse yet, try to make sense of an itemized bill from an emergency room visit or hospital stay. Recent studies clearly demonstrate that most individuals are unable to correctly "translate" this information.

Finally, the resources available to assess the quality of a medical service or product are frequently absent, inferior, or too difficult to understand. Such resources *are* available to consumers but deciding which are reliable and unbiased is a great challenge. Far too many of the consumer rating resources on the internet for doctors, clinics, and hospitals are funded by the doctors or facilities being rated, which raises obvious concerns regarding bias and reliability. The issue of patient testimonials in these resources also must be viewed with caution. There is potential for fraud and abuse on both the negative and positive side. Unethical individuals wanting to boost the rating of a provider or facility can post any number of glowing testimonials under different names. On the other hand, someone with a grudge could do the same with negative postings.

Yet even when these resources are found to be unbiased and reliable, there are numerous independent scientific reviews that consistently find that these ratings and reviews from patients primarily measure such things as waiting times and bedside manner. These measures are certainly important and useful in making consumer decisions in health care.

However, they do not address arguably the most important measure, which is the actual quality of the medical care provided. For instance, there are no consumer resources reporting on physicians that can reliably measure either the accuracy of diagnoses being made or whether treatment recommendations are based on the best current scientific evidence. Due to the complexity of being able to acquire and track this information, it is not likely this information will be available soon.

Overcoming the numerous anti-consumerism elements of our current healthcare system is indeed a formidable task. The political courage necessary to bring about meaningful health insurance reform seems to be lacking, and the pressure that should force the healthcare industry to provide consumers with transparency and up-front pricing information will take time. Chapter 16 will address some short- and medium-term solutions to the perplexing problem.

CHAPTER 14

The Role of Overuse in the Misallocation of Healthcare Resources

One of the most perplexing causes of the high cost of medical care is the misallocation of resources in healthcare delivery that results in a tremendous amount of waste and inefficiency. This occurs at both ends of the spectrum in terms of both overuse and underuse of medical services and products. In addition to the dollar cost, there is the potential for this misallocated health care to create adverse health events, with the inevitable result of physical and emotional damage.

Overuse of medical services involves diagnostic and/or treatment activities that have one or more of these three characteristics:

- No proven benefit
- Proven harmful results
- Better alternatives (including no action at all).

Underuse involves the failure to take advantage of healthcare measures that are based on the best current scientific evidence and have proven health benefits. This issue is the subject of the next chapter.

Both extremes represent a failure in healthcare delivery. It may be a failure on the part of healthcare providers in making the correct recommendations or a refusal of healthcare consumers to take proper medical advice when offered. In either case, the result is generally unfavorable and sometimes dangerous. Although the goal of attaining 100 percent "appropriate care" is unrealistic, a significant reduction from currently unacceptable levels of overuse and underuse is not.

A recent respected study by the Institute of Medicine attempted to put an annual dollar amount on the waste associated with this misallocation of resources. The Institute published the following figures:[49]

- $210 billion for unnecessary medical services
- $190 billion for excessive administrative costs
- $130 billion for inefficiently delivered services
- $105 billion for overpriced services
- $75 billion for fraud
- $55 billion for missed prevention opportunities.

This totals $765 billion and represents over 20 percent of total spending on health care. Overuse of medical resources is prevalent throughout all areas of health care, and the following information provides insight into some representative examples of this serious problem.

---

49 "Antibiotic Use in Outpatient Settings, 2017." Centers for Disease Control and Prevention. Last modified August 8, 2019. https://www.cdc.gov/antibiotic-use/stewardship-report/outpatient.html.

Perhaps the most common example is the over-prescription of antibiotics, which was touched on in chapter 10. There are currently over 100 antibiotics available to healthcare providers. Antibiotics have rightfully been viewed as miracle drugs since their discovery and development over the last number of decades. They have helped to cure countless serious infections which at one time had no effective treatment and have therefore saved millions of lives.

However, the evidence is overwhelming that there are major difficulties when it comes to the inappropriate use of these agents. This has led to serious problems that offset some of the amazing benefits of appropriate use of antibiotics. There are at least three major adverse results from antibiotic overuse:

- The pure waste of the financial cost of the drug itself that amounts to millions of dollars annually
- The potential for serious drug side effects that are not rare and can be serious to the point of causing death
- The grave issue of fostering resistance to antibiotics.

It is not complicated to explain how antibiotic resistance occurs. Our body's immune system has a remarkable capacity to fend off infections. However, there are cases in which this system does not work effectively. This is when antibiotic use should be considered. Antibiotics work through assisting our natural immune system by killing, or at least disabling, the microbes (bacteria, viruses, etc.) that cause disease. When everything goes well, the infection is cured.

The undesirable result of antibiotic resistance occurs when some of these targeted microbes "survive" the antibiotic used in the infection battle. They then have the remarkable capacity to develop mutations in their DNA that render the antibiotic ineffective the next time it is used against this strain of microbe. This leads to the necessity of developing stronger antibiotics to deal with this resistance. All this sets up a vicious cycle leading to more and more microbial resistance and the development of stronger and more potent antibiotics. These stronger drugs come with a much higher price tag and tend to have more potent and dangerous side effects. This is a cycle that must be interrupted.

These statistics describe the scope of the problem:[50]

- The CDC Source issued a report indicating that in 2015, 269 million antibiotic prescriptions were dispensed and at least 30% (over 80 million) were unnecessary.
- There are more than two million infections caused by antibiotic-resistant microbes annually and 23,000 of these end in death.
- Antibiotic resistance is estimated to cost our nation over $2 billion each year.
- The rate of antibiotic-resistant infections doubled from 2002 to 2014.

Most of the over-prescription of antibiotics comes from physicians issuing the prescription when:

- The diagnosis is incorrect, such as when a runny nose and cough that are caused by an allergy are treated as an infection
- There is a bacterial infection, and the best option is NOT to prescribe an antibiotic but to let the body's

---

50 Tavernise, Sabrina. "Antibiotic-Resistant Infections Lead to 23,000 Deaths a Year, C.D.C. Finds." The New York Times, September 16, 2013. https://www.nytimes.com/2013/09/17/health/cdc-report-finds-23000-deaths-a-year-from-antibiotic-resistant-infections.html.

- own immune system work, as it does very well in many cases of uncomplicated sinus, ear, and bronchial infections
- There is an infection, but the microbe causing the infection is not susceptible to antibiotics; for example, the majority of common upper respiratory infections are caused by a virus and should never be treated with amoxicillin, a "Z-Pack," or similar antibiotics that are only effective against bacteria
- There is a bacterial infection that is serious enough to warrant an antibiotic, but the incorrect antibiotic (often one that is more potent than required) is prescribed instead of the recommended first-line antibiotic that generally has the lesser chance of creating resistance.

The blame for this must be borne primarily by the healthcare providers that are writing the inappropriate antibiotic prescriptions. They have the prime responsibility of making the correct diagnosis and recommendation for whether antibiotic treatment is appropriate. However, patients must also share in this to a lesser degree, as many studies have shown that physicians are frequently pressured by patients to give antibiotics for almost any condition that appears to be an infection. A trustworthy physician must resist this pressure and use such an encounter to educate and "first, do no harm."

There is evidence that recent efforts directed at both healthcare providers and patients to reduce inappropriate antibiotic prescribing is having some positive effects. Several studies have shown as much as a 13 percent decline in the prescribing of broad-spectrum antibiotics, which are those most associated with bacterial resistance.[51]

---

51 "Antibiotic Prescription Fill Rates Declining in the U.S." Blue Cross Blue Shield. Last modified August 24, 2017.

It should be noted that antibiotics are by no means the only drugs being overprescribed and contributing to waste of healthcare resources. This problem exists with almost all categories of drugs. It occurs across all age groups, but it is especially serious in the senior population. The term for this is poly-pharmacology, and the extent of the problem is demonstrated by the fact that 40 percent of seniors are taking multiple drugs.[52] It is factual that many seniors have multiple chronic health conditions, and there are legitimate reasons for some individuals to require multiple medications. It is common for these medications to come from several, if not multiple, healthcare providers. However, avoiding harm in such circumstances requires ironclad communication between all prescribing providers with very careful regular monitoring and periodic medication reconciliation to check for necessity, effectiveness, side effects, and drug-drug interactions. Unfortunately, this communication and monitoring is too frequently lacking.

While on this subject of misallocation of resources in the area of pharmacology, we should address the issue of the overuse of brand-name drugs that have equally effective, and much less expensive, generic alternatives. There was a time when the quality control for generic drugs was not adequate, but that is no longer the case. While there are cases where the brand-name drug is more suitable than a generic equivalent, these are in the minority.

---

    https://www.bcbs.com/the-health-of-america/reports/antibiotic-prescription-rates-declining-in-the-US.

52   Charlesworth, Christina J., Ellen Smit, David S. Lee, Fatimah Alramadhan, and Michelle C. Odden. "Polypharmacy Among Adults Aged 65 Years and Older in the United States: 1988–2010." J Gerontol A Biol Sci Med Sci. 70, no. 8 (August 2015): 989-95. https://doi.org/10.1093/gerona/glv013.

A recent report indicated that for 2017, the use of generic drugs over their brand-name counterparts saved $265 billion.[53] There is a positive trend toward ever greater use of generic equivalents (including over-the-counter medications), and studies indicate that billions of additional dollars can be saved if this continues.

The next example of overuse of resources involves the inappropriate use of imaging, including routine X-rays, CAT scans, MRIs, and PET scans. The use of high-tech imaging is one of the fastest growing areas in health care. There is no question as to the great benefit of appropriate use of these technologies in the diagnosis and treatment of serious diseases.

However, numerous studies indicate that a significant percentage of these tests provide no useful benefit, result in huge financial waste, and carry some grave risks for patients. The risks include excessive radiation exposure (especially CAT scans) with the accompanying increased risk for cancer. Some of these tests require the use of contrast agents that can cause serious allergic reactions. Then there are the adverse consequences of false positive results leading to additional testing and treatment, with the resulting additional financial costs and anxiety. A great example is imaging for the very common problem of low back pain. This was described in some detail in chapter 10 and will not be repeated here but is worth reviewing.

Another common example of overuse of healthcare resources is unnecessary surgery. Just as with antibiotics and other pharmaceuticals, there have been amazing advances in surgery that have extended the quality and length of life for millions. However, there are many common surgeries

---

53   "2018 Generic Drug Access and Savings Report." Association f or Accessible Medicines. https://accessiblemeds.org/2018-generic-drug-access-and-savings-report.

performed annually that have no proven benefit and are avoidable.

One of the most common is unnecessary surgery for low back pain that is tied directly to the previous topic of overuse of imaging. Similarly, studies have shown that many patients with a damaged knee meniscus have no better outcome with arthroscopic surgery than if they elect to do physical therapy.[54] There are many more examples, but every unnecessary surgery shares the potential for complications from infection, pain, and anesthetic accidents that can be fatal.

The advent of PAP smears in 1940s revolutionized health care for women. Widespread adoption of screening with PAP smears has resulted in cervical cancer dropping from first to thirteenth place as a cause of death in women.[55] Yet following the same trend as with drugs and surgery, there is currently a large degree of overuse of the PAP test that has financial and emotional costs.[56]

For most of the last half of the 20th century, the standard recommendation was to get a PAP test every year. Recommendations for screening have changed in recent years due to an increased understanding of how cervical can-

---

54 "An Epidemic of Unnecessary Surgeries." Health Link Medical Center. https://healthlinkcenter.com/epidemic-of-unnecessary-surgeries/.

55 Safaeian, Mahboobeh, Diane Solomon, and Philip E. Castle. "Cervical Cancer Prevention - Cervical Screening: Science in Evolution." Obstetrics and Gynecology Clinics of North America 34, no. 4 (December 2007): 739-60. https://doi.org/10.1016/j.ogc.2007.09.004.

56 Almeida, C M., M A. Rodriguez, S Skootsky, and J Pregler. "Cervical Cancer Screening Overuse and Underuse: Patient and Physician Factors." American Journal of Managed Care 19, no. 6 (June 2013): 482-9. https://www.ncbi.nlm.nih.gov/pubmed/23844709.

cer develops, advances in the technology of the PAP smear, and additional tests that can detect cervical cancer at an early stage. For the majority of women aged 21-35 that are of average risk for cervical cancer, the PAP smear should be done every three years. For most women under age 21 and over age 65, PAP smears may not be needed.[57] To be clear, there are exceptions to this for women at higher than average risk, and this must be determined for each woman individually.

As in all incidences of overuse of medical services, unnecessary PAP tests carry the element of financial waste. Yet the most significant cost is the avoidable stress and anxiety the women who get a "false positive" abnormality report are subjected to, followed by additional costly testing and the added emotional stress of waiting for the results.

A very troublesome area of overuse is found in the practice of certain routine screening tests for the disease in persons without any symptoms. As with all the previous overuse examples, there are valuable routine screening tests that have great benefits, such as cancer screening for breast and colon cancer. However, other routine testing such as ECGs, chest X-rays, and simple blood counts that commonly occur with annual physicals and preoperative exams have been shown to be of little to no value but carry an annual cost into the billions of dollars.[58]

Of special concern is the growing practice of companies offering a group of medical screening tests for car-

---

57 "Cervical Cancer Screening FAQ085." The American College of Obstetricians and Gynecologists. Last modified September 2017. https://www.acog.org/Patients/FAQs/Cervical-Cancer-Screening?IsMobileSet=false.
58 Kale, Minal S., Tara F. Bishop, and Alex D. Federman. "'Top 5' Lists Top $5 Billion." JAMA Internal Medicine 171, no. 20 (November 2011): 1858-59. https://doi.org/doi:10.1001/archinternmed.2011.501.

diovascular disease and osteoporosis directly to the public. These are offered at a relatively affordable cost (usually under $150) and are advertised to detect serious disease conditions before symptoms occur. The are several problems with these screenings. The most serious is that there are no major scientific organizations that endorse them. The reason for this is that the preponderance of evidence at this time is that these screenings do more harm than good overall.[59]

The companies offering these screenings cite numerous anecdotal examples of success in detecting a serious problem unknown to the patient. Yet the best evidence is that for every person benefiting from early detection there are far more people that undergo needless additional unnecessary testing and treatment resulting from false positives in these bulk screening tests. This causes needless suffering from the stress and anxiety created. There is also the additional danger of having a false negative test result from these bulk screenings. This may cause a false sense of security that can result in a person later ignoring symptoms that should be investigated.

Finally, there is a concern over the quality of both the equipment used in these screening and the accuracy of the interpretation of the results.[60] The bottom line is that the best approach to screening for disease should come after a frank discussion with an ethical healthcare professional resulting in full knowledge of the pros and cons of each individual test.

---

59   "By the Way, Doctor: Should I be Tested at Life Line Screening?" Harvard Health. https://www.health.harvard.edu/newsletter_article/By_the_way_doctor_Should_I_be_tested_at_Life_Line_Screening.

60   "18 Million Avoidable Hospital Emergency Department Visits Add $32 Billion in Costs to the Health Care System Each Year." United Heath Group. Last modified 2019. https://www.unitedhealthgroup.com/content/dam/UHG/PDF/2019/UHG-Avoidable-ED-Visits.pdf.

This is lacking in many of these direct-to-consumer bulk screenings.

Another particularly important overuse healthcare activity is visiting the emergency room (ER) for treatment of conditions that are not truly emergencies. It is estimated that two-thirds of the 27 million ER visits by patients with private insurance in the U.S. are avoidable and should have been in a primary care setting.[61] This not only creates a huge financial waste, but it also diverts medical staff and resources away from those patients with true emergencies that are in need of immediate, perhaps lifesaving, attention.

There are many more examples of overuse of healthcare resources but covering them all is beyond the scope of this book. However, there is one additional problem in overuse that deserves mention here. This involves the highly sensitive issue of end-of-life care. There has been extensive research on this subject that reveals these facts and statistics:

- Medicare spends a large percent of its budget on health care in the last year of life[62]
- This money spent often has a minimal impact on extending the length of life and can decrease the quality of life through complications and side effects of treatment[63]

---

61 The Cost of Dying: End-of-Life Care. Directed by Andy Court, CBS, 2010. DVD.
62 Smith, Alexander, Ellen McCarthy, Ellen Weber, Irena S. Cenzer, and John Boscardin. "Half Of Older Americans Seen In Emergency Department In Last Month Of Life; Most Admitted To Hospital, And Many Die There." Health Aff (Millwood) 31, no. 6 (June 2012): 1277-85. https://doi.org/10.1377/hlthaff.2011.0922.
63 Amadeo, Kimberly. "The Rising Cost of Health Care by Year and Its Causes." The Balance. Last modified January

- Patients average almost 30 office visits in the last six months of life[64]
- In the last month of life:

  — 50% of patients end up in the emergency room
  — 33% are admitted to ICU
  — 25% undergo surgery.[65]

Everyone has the right to expect our healthcare system to make every *reasonable* effort to prolong life. In every poll taken on the subject of end-of-life wishes, the majority of individuals express the desire to die peacefully at home and not in a hospital. Specifically, most people express the desire not to be kept alive on machines or with heroic efforts resulting in a life with little or no quality. The above statistics indicate that this is too often not the case.

This end-of-life care issue is one problem for which there are available solutions that should be implemented by every individual. These are detailed in the final chapter.

14, 2020. https://www.thebalance.com/causes-of-rising-health care-costs-4064878.

64 Amadeo, Kimberly. "The Rising Cost of Health Care by Year and Its Causes."

65 Amadeo, Kimberly. "The Rising Cost of Health Care by Year and Its Causes."

CHAPTER 15

The Role of Underuse in the Misallocation of Healthcare Resources

At the other end of the misallocation spectrum is the issue of underuse of healthcare services, which occurs whenever:

- Healthcare providers fail to recommend preventive medicine activities or diagnostic and treatment measures that are based on the best current scientific evidence (known as evidence-based medicine).
- Patients fail, refuse, or are unable to take advantage of evidence-based medicine (preventive or treatment).

There is no good excuse for healthcare providers contributing to this problem of underuse by failing or neglecting to present the best evidenced-based options for their patients. It unfortunately implies incompetency, complacency, poor communication skills, or negligence. This underscores the necessity for healthcare consumers to develop the trusting relationship with their healthcare provider(s) that was the focus of the first 10 chapters of this book.

The issue of patients not taking advantage of evidenced-based medicine is more complex. While healthcare providers have firm professional, ethical, and legal obligations to provide the correct best-evidence options to their patients, patients may have understandable reasons for not seeking or accepting what is currently considered sound medical advice. The most unfortunate of these reasons would be lack of access to health care and/or financial inability to pay. There are also individuals that may avoid traditional medical care on the basis of religious or other personal beliefs. People who have personally experienced or witnessed a bad outcome with medical treatment may have an understandable mistrust of the medical profession. Yet while the autonomy and the personal choice of each patient must be respected, there is strong evidence that many patients suffer needlessly by refusing to heed sound medical advice. This also confers a large financial burden on society.

As with overuse, there are too many examples to be able to cover them all in this book. However, the following information should be sufficient to demonstrate the scope of the problem. Some areas of underuse are the other side of the coin of overuse. For example:

- As described in the previous chapter, PAP smears are being done too frequently for many women, but there are also women who do not get them at all or not frequently enough to get the benefit of early detection of cervical cancer.
- The practice of visiting the emergency room for minor problems is contrasted with the failure to go to the emergency room promptly enough to prevent complications, such as attributing chest pain

to "indigestion" when it is actually a sign of a heart attack.

A very common area of underuse involves low rates of recommended immunizations. Vaccinations have been scientifically shown without any doubt to have far greater individual and societal health benefits than risks. Although there are other factors, such as better hygiene, that have caused a decrease in diseases that have been targeted by vaccination, there is no serious opposition to the fact that immunizations have been the major reasons for statistics such as:[66]

- In 1950 in the U.S., there were over 300,000 cases of measles; in 2017 this number was 468
- In 1950 in the U.S., there were over 33,000 cases of polio with almost 2,000 deaths and thousands of children and adults left with permanent paralysis; there has not been more than one case of polio per year since 2,000 and no deaths
- There are similar numbers for many once-common childhood and adult diseases for which there are now recommended vaccines.

However, before proceeding with this subject, it would be useful to address the unfortunate controversy surrounding vaccinations. There is a small, but very vocal, anti-vaccination (anti-vax) movement that is contributing to an alarming resurgence of serious diseases that were at one point under good control or virtually eradicated. It is a fact that there are

---

[66] "Reported Cases and Deaths from Vaccine Preventable Diseases, United States, 1950-2005." Centers for Disease Control and Prevention. Last modified May 2019. https://www.cdc.gov/vaccines/pubs/pinkbook/downloads/appendices/E/reported-cases.pdf.

instances of serious complications that have resulted from currently recommended vaccinations. Yet these events are comparatively rare compared to the numbers of individuals that are spared from the disability, or even death, that results from many diseases prevented by immunization. A typical example of this would be whooping cough or pertussis. In the 1940s, over 200,000 children suffered from whooping cough and over 9,000 died from the condition annually. In the 1980s the number of cases dropped to an average of less than 2,000 per year, with single-digit deaths per year.

In the last 10-15 years, reports of a rare, but serious, neurological complication from the whooping cough vaccine have been widely published. However, those reports often neglect to balance that information with the well-known history of the above successes of the vaccine. As a result, great numbers of children are failing to receive the whooping cough vaccine, and now the annual cases are as high as 40,000, with around 20 deaths.[67]

There is no doubt that the parents who decided to withhold the whooping cough vaccine for their children were well-intentioned. Most of them were likely not aware of the lifesaving facts of the vaccine or the potential severity of this disease that many of them had never encountered. However, they were very likely, and understandably, fearful and concerned about the serious, but quite rare, neurological complications emphasized by the anti-vax voices. It is without question sound parenting practice to be fully informed in these matters. However, this requires a careful and objective assessment of all the facts and evidence.

The whooping cough vaccine story is a situation in which the loudest voices can drown out the clear evidence

---

67 "Whooping Cough (Pertussis)." National Foundation for Infectious Diseases. https://www.nfid.org/infectious-diseases/pertussis-whooping-cough/.

that a child is far more likely to be helped than harmed by the vaccine. Much of the responsibility for this lies at the feet of the medical profession that has not effectively and compassionately conveyed the scientific evidence to parents. In addition, the media establishment has a duty to be more thorough and balanced in reporting on such issues and less concerned with sensational, attention-grabbing headlines when lives are at stake.

Another similar scenario involves the issue of the concern that autism is caused by vaccines. This tragic story began primarily in 1998 with the publication of an article in the highly prestigious medical journal, the *Lancet*. In summary, this article suggested a link between the MMR (measles, mumps, and rubella) vaccine and autism. This was picked up by media outlets and the result was a marked decrease in understandably frightened parents allowing their children to obtain the MMR vaccine. Subsequent measles outbreaks in both the U.S. and Britain are linked to these events.

In a matter of a few years, most of the 12 authors of the *Lancet* article disassociated themselves with the findings in the article. In 2010, the *Lancet* also retracted the entire article. The British medical establishment "struck off" the main author of the article for serious professional misconduct. Many subsequent respected scientific studies have refuted any connection between autism and the MMR vaccine.[68]

There have been similar concerns expressed about mercury-containing preservatives in vaccines causing autism. This has garnered a lot of attention in the media and is championed in anti-vax circles. Although virtually all vaccines have eliminated such preservatives, there are those that continue to

---

68 Rao, T S., and C Andrade. "The MMR vaccine and autism: Sensation, refutation, retraction, and fraud." Indian Journal of Psychiatry 53, no. 2 (April 2011): 95-96. https://doi.org/10.4103/0019-5545.82529.

make this claim. There have been numerous respected studies of these preservatives that have found no link to autism.[69] However, it is very easy to understand how parents of a child with autism, or parents wanting to do anything to prevent autism in their child, would be influenced by misinformation.

Preventing such incidents of dissemination and acceptance of misinformation will require a joint effort on the part of all involved. The scientific research community needs to strengthen its oversight of published findings to regain the trust of the public. The medical profession must do better with conveying the risks and benefits of every medical decision and consistently engage patients in true shared decision-making.

While the healthcare consumer needs to be vigilant and able to make tough and informed decisions, he or she must attempt not to fall prey to sensational media headlines reporting on unproven pseudoscience. There must also be an awareness that misinformation can be driven by often well-intentioned individuals and groups that are understandably motivated by the emotion of personal tragedy rather than the best available scientific evidence.

However, in spite of all the problems surrounding immunizations, the facts in this area are overwhelmingly on the side of the mainstream view. This view acknowledges the valid concerns about the risks of vaccinations but understands that the vast majority of individuals benefit greatly from receiving the currently recommended immunizations. Before leaving this subject, the following are a few more statistics regarding the health and financial benefits of vaccines:

- In 1994, a program to fund and encourage childhood immunizations was launched. These are the

---

69   "Science Summary: CDC Studies on Thimerosal in Vaccines." Centers for Disease Control and Prevention. https://www.cdc.gov/vaccinesafety/pdf/cdcstudiesonvaccinesandautism.pdf.

modeled results for the 79 million children born during 1994-2013 that achieved vaccination rates of over 90% as a result of this program:[70]

- Prevention of 322 million illnesses
- Prevention of 21 million hospitalizations
- Prevention of 732,000 premature deaths
- A net savings of $295 billion in direct costs and $1.38 trillion in total societal costs.

✍ These are the projected financial costs (aside from the human suffering) of non-vaccination in adults for four common vaccine-preventable diseases:[71]

- Total annual cost = $8.95 billion; cost of each disease individually:
    - Influenza – $5.9 billion
    - Shingles – $1.86 billion
    - HPV (cause of cervical cancer and others) – $333 million
    - Hepatitis B – $173 million.

---

70 Whitney, Cynthia G., Fangjun Zhou, James Singleton, and Anne Schuchat. "Benefits from Immunization During the Vaccines for Children Program Era — United States, 1994–2013." Morbidity and Mortality Weekly Report 63, no. 16 (April 25, 2014): 352-55. https://www.ncbi.nlm.nih.gov/pmc/articles/PMC4584777/.

71 Ozawa, Sachiko, Allison Portnoy, Hiwote Getaneh, Samantha Clark, and Maria Knoll. "Modeling The Economic Burden Of Adult Vaccine-Preventable Diseases In The United States." Health Affairs 35, no. 11. https://doi.org/doi.org/10.1377/hlthaff.2016.0462.

Perhaps the most widespread, and arguably the most important, problem with healthcare underuse is the lack of promoting and implementing the wisest lifestyle choices affecting physical, mental, and spiritual health. This failure is shared by both a healthcare system that currently puts far too few resources toward this critical aspect of preventive medicine and by individuals who make self-destructive lifestyle decisions. However, the importance and impact of this problem may become even more clear with information on the costs in both human suffering and dollars.

There are many examples of poor lifestyle choices in America. These choices are major risk factors for the development of the most common causes of premature death and disability from potentially preventable disorders, including heart disease, diabetes, arthritis, and cancer. The following are examples of three of the most common of these risk factors with particularly alarming statistics:

- Smoking[72]

    - Smoking and other tobacco use kills over 480,000 Americans every year
    - Thousands more live with disabling lung disease caused by smoking
    - The financial cost of tobacco-related illness is over $300 billion annually. It includes:

        - $170 billion in medical care
        - $156 billion in lost worker productivity.

---

72 "Tobacco-Related Mortality." Centers for Disease Control and Prevention. Last modified 2014. https://www.cdc.gov/tobacco/data_statistics/fact_sheets/health_effects/tobacco_related_mortality/index.htm.

- Poor diet, lack of physical activity, and obesity[73]

    - 22% of all deaths (over 600,000) in the U.S. are linked to these factors
    - The financial burden to the U.S.:

        - Low-level physical activity – $117 billion
        - Obesity – over $150 billion[74]

- Alcohol and other drug abuse[75]

    - 5.6% of all deaths (over 150,000) in the U.S.
    - Abuse of alcohol and both illicit drugs and prescription drugs cost the U.S. over $500 **billion** including direct healthcare costs, lost productivity, vehicular accidents, and criminal justice expenses.

The total human suffering and financial costs of just these three poor lifestyle choice examples is staggering. As mentioned above, the source of this problem lies with both the healthcare delivery system and the healthcare consumer.

---

73   Carlson, S A., E K. Adams, Z Yang, and J E. Fulton. "Percentage of Deaths Associated With Inadequate Physical Activity in the United States." Preventing Chronic Disease 15 (March 29, 2018). https://doi.org/doi.org/10.5888/pcd18.170354.

74   "Obesity: Facts, Figures, Guidelines." West Virginia Department of Health and Human Resources. Last modified December 2002. https://www.wvdhhr.org/bph/oehp/obesity/mortality.htm.

75   "Economic Cost of Substance Abuse in the United States." Recovery Centers of America. https://recoverycentersofamerica.com/economic-cost-substance-abuse/.

It follows that the solution must come from changes in both of these contributors.

There is virtually universal agreement that the current healthcare delivery system is heavily weighted toward diagnosis and treatment compared to resources directed at prevention of disease. There are historical, financial, and human nature factors that are behind this imbalance. In the late 19th and early 20th centuries, as medicine began to change from leeches and bloodletting to a modern, scientifically based profession, some of the earliest successes were purely preventive. Improvements in public health were at the forefront of these achievements. Advances in simple, low-tech measures such as clean water, food safety, personal hygiene, and workplace safety made a great difference in both quality and length of life.

As important as these preventive achievements were, they became vastly overshadowed in the mid-to-late 20th century by amazing treatment and diagnostic advances in the fields of surgery, pharmaceuticals, and high-tech imaging. This imbalance persists today. Although there has been some improvement, the current curriculum for medical students remains heavily weighted toward treatment. It is therefore not surprising that this is the focus of new doctors in their medical practices upon graduation. This is reinforced by the current system of insurance reimbursement for healthcare services and products. The amounts paid for diagnostic and treatment activities are generally much higher than those for preventive services.

Finally, there is the human nature factor. For patients requiring medical care, there is too often a natural attraction and fascination for high-tech imaging. There is a similar attitude toward opting for surgery or taking potent drugs instead of taking preventive action that may involve making difficult changes in lifestyle. Two such common examples include treatment of high cholesterol and marked obesity. For high cholesterol, many individuals opt to take a daily pill instead of making a concerted effort to change eating and physical activity habits. Similarly, many people opt for gastric surgery for obesity in spite of the dangers of these surgeries compared to very low-risk lifestyle changes in nutrition and exercise.

Unfortunately, too many physicians will give into, or even promote, these approaches as they experience the common futility of advocating for the non-drug lifestyle changes in diet and exercise. These same human nature challenges exist for approaches to many other common medical conditions such as diabetes and high blood pressure. The primary solution to this underuse issue will be addressed in the final chapter.

CHAPTER 16

Strategies for Coping with High Healthcare Costs

The previous three chapters provided explanations for some of the major causes of high healthcare costs. Some of these have no immediate or short-term solutions. However, this chapter will describe some of the definite opportunities for positive change in many of the other problem areas. Some of these proposed solutions will require substantial collaborative societal efforts and political courage and therefore may take some time to realize. Yet, many of the following opportunities can be implemented with both short and long-term benefits in physical, mental, and spiritual, and financial well-being. These proposed solutions and reforms will be addressed in the approximate order they were addressed in the last three chapters.

Chapter 12 concentrated on four problems driving high healthcare costs in the areas of supply and demand. Two of these included the increase in the senior population (demand) and the decrease in the percentage of younger persons (supply). There are, of course, no practical solutions to these population factors. However, there are definite solutions for the other two issues of a projected shortage of over 122,000 physicians (supply) and the epidemic of chronic diseases (demand). The chronic disease solutions will be dealt with in more detail in the section below addressing the overuse and underuse of healthcare resources from chapters 14 and 15.

It is imperative that the looming physician shortage problem be resolved. There are solutions, but they are complex and require:

- An increase in both medical school class sizes and post-graduate residency training positions in teaching hospitals
- Remedies for physician burnout and early retirement
- The remaining shortage must be handled through a team approach with highly trained non-physician providers and patient self-care aided by technology and telemedicine.

There has been some progress in producing more medical school graduates, with an increase of about 30 percent in medical school positions in the past few years. However, these additional medical school graduates must have post-graduate residency positions for the additional training required before entering practice. (there are a few exceptions to this, but medical school graduates without a residency have many limitations and frequently cannot obtain hospital privileges or receive reimbursement from insurance companies). There has been only a 10 percent increase in additional residency positions, which falls far short of what is required for the 30 percent increase in medical students.[76,77] There is an awareness of this deficiency and there appears to be optimism that the funding to increase these residency positions will be met. However, even when this does occur, it will be insufficient to deal with the projected shortage. [78]

The shortfall must be made up on two fronts. The first is to slow down the rate of early retirement of currently practicing physicians by effectively dealing with the issue of burnout and professional dissatisfaction. The American Medical Association and many state medical societies have begun to offer anti-burnout programs and other resources to their members. There are also active lobbying efforts being directed at state and federal lawmakers to streamline and, where appropriate, eliminate burdensome regulations, paperwork, and red tape that have not proven to live up to their original goals of better health care. The action that would have the most impact would be to remove insurance companies and government bureaucrats from the medical decision-making process as much as possible.

Second, we must expand the role of highly trained, non-physician healthcare providers, such as nurse practitioners, physician assistants, physical therapists, nurse educators, psychologists, etc. Some physician professional groups

---

76 Japsen, Bruce. "U.S. Doctor Shortage Could Hit 90,000 By 2025." Forbes, March 3, 2015. https://www.forbes.com/sites/brucejapsen/2015/03/03/u-s-doctor-shortage-could-hit-90000-by-2025/#3919ae2b9285.

77 "The Role of GME Funding in Addressing the Physician Shortage." Association of American Medical Colleges. https://www.aamc.org/news-insights/gme.

78 "U.S. Medical School Enrollment Surpasses Expansion Goal." American Association of Medical Colleges. Last modified July 25, 2019. https://www.aamc.org/news-insights/press-releases/us-medical-school-enrollment-surpasses-expansion-goal.

and societies have raised objections to this expansion with concerns about non-physicians taking on responsibilities beyond their ability. However, experience to date has shown that these healthcare providers can add great benefit to direct patient care (and ease the current workload and stress of physicians) without compromising quality of care if the distribution of duties and scope of practices are clearly defined.

It has been our professional and personal experience that a board-certified family nurse practitioner can competently perform 75-80 percent of the daily duties of a primary care physician. These non-physician providers consistently perform as high or higher than physicians in surveys of patient satisfaction. Forward-thinking physicians are embracing, and not resisting, these highly valuable assets.

In this same realm, are the opportunities that lie in the area of increasing patient self-care in the age of the internet and advances in technology. Although technology often is a two-edged sword, and there is truth to the old saying that "a little knowledge can be a dangerous thing," the potential benefits of patients assuming a greater role in their own health care are enormous.

Healthcare has fallen far behind other industries such as banking, shopping, travel, and communication when it comes to using technology to allow individuals to perform functions that were once exclusive to professionals. This is slowly changing, and there are increasing examples of this as seen with home monitoring of blood pressure, blood sugar, and blood thinners. There are also over-the-counter diagnostic tests for pregnancy, urinary tract infections, etc.

The expansion of electronic medical records and scheduling resources currently allows some patients to schedule their own appointments, view test results, and communicate electronically with their providers. For a few uncomplicated, but common, medical conditions such as strep throat, influenza, or urinary tract infection, it is not difficult to imagine a patient being able to self-diagnose and self-treat without direct involvement of a healthcare provider. Also, with the increasing availability and accuracy of home testing equipment, it is possible for patients to have more involvement in the routine care of common chronic conditions such as high blood pressure and diabetes. This could reduce the number of routine office visits, resulting in cost savings and freeing up office time for other issues that clearly require face-to-face time with a healthcare provider.

Finally, telemedicine holds the promise of bringing needed resources to remote and underserved communities. There are many examples of this currently in practice. Rural emergency rooms can access specialists in real-time to manage problems that once formally required expensive and often dangerous patient transfers. There are dermatologists that can make accurate diagnoses remotely by receiving high-quality images of skin conditions. There is even the possibility of "telesurgery," which permits a surgeon to perform a procedure without being physically present with the patient. This primarily robotic activity is in its infancy, but it does seem to have great potential to become an important part of the solution to the pending physician shortage.

Solving the problems that were described in chapter 13 regarding the lack of healthcare consumerism in today's environment is a definite challenge. Meaningful progress for this problem across our whole society will only be possible with major reforms in the U.S. medical economic system. The current system creates barriers between the healthcare consumer and the information the consumer needs to make the best financial decisions for this very expensive and essential "commodity." The information needed includes up-front transparency and accuracy of pricing for healthcare goods and services and reliable quality ratings for providers and facilities. Additional reforms are needed to provide insurance portability and greater freedom of choice of providers and healthcare facilities.

However, even though the current political and social polarization in this country is an obstacle for these needed reforms, there are steps that individuals and groups can and should take now. Hopefully, the first 10 chapters of this book will have provided a foundation for this. If a patient has a good shared decision-making relationship with a trustworthy primary healthcare provider, this can serve as a home base for basic medical care and can be a reliable clearinghouse for medical needs beyond primary care.

This requires patients to be informed and assertive in requesting accurate and up-front pricing at the point of care. Armed with the information in chapter 13 regarding all the potential anti-consumerism built into the current system, patients should be able to keep third-party payers (private or government) from obscuring the actual costs. This will be easier for the non-emergency, high-volume services such as imaging, elective outpatient procedures, and childbirth.

This effort will be enhanced with a trusted primary care provider who is willing to move out of his or her comfort zone and take on a likely unfamiliar and perhaps uncomfortable role of financial advocacy in this process. It will also require some courage on the part of healthcare providers who must acknowledge that the current fee-for-service system that rewards volume must be replaced, at least in part, by a patient-centered reimbursement system. This system would pay for the delivery of "bundled" services and be tied to the achievement of predefined outcomes. There will always be resistance to such major change, but the momentum does seem to be moving in this direction.

Perhaps the greatest opportunities for a consumer to control personal healthcare costs involve avoiding the overuse or underuse of medical care as covered in chapters 14 and 15. This is best termed "appropriate care." Taking complete advantage of these opportunities requires action on two levels:

- Personal:
  - Wise lifestyle choices
  - Self-care
  - Advanced directives.

- Professional:
  - Informed shared decision-making with a trusted healthcare provider
  - Using reliable resources to verify healthcare provider recommendations (trust but verify).

On the personal level, a major factor in obtaining appropriate medical care is the decision to make wise lifestyle choices. These can minimize the amount of professional medical care needed by preventing disease and injury. The decisions each individual makes regarding the care of body, mind, and spirit have an enormous impact on a person's overall health. It is hard to argue the fact that one's most precious asset is good health. Fortunately, basic health maintenance generally requires no special training or assistance from other individuals. There are simple fundamentals that include eating a balanced diet, getting regular physical activity, avoiding toxic or addictive substances and behaviors, and providing for mental and spiritual nurturing.

However, just because something is simple does not mean it is necessarily easy. The above health maintenance fundamentals are indeed simple. However, the fact that they may require tough choices and decisions in everyday human behavior may make them difficult to carry out. Nutrition is perhaps the best example of this.

JUDSON HENDERSON, M.D
PATRICIA HENDERSON, FNP-BC

Most Americans have an abundant and relatively inexpensive food supply at their disposal, including highly nutritious choices. Ironically, far too many individuals make fast and easy choices that are high in calories and low in nutritional value. Once these choices become a habit, it becomes very difficult to change. One result of this is an epidemic of obesity that is a major contributor to the rise in chronic diseases such as diabetes and high blood pressure. This in turn increases the incidence of cardiovascular disease, which is the number one cause of premature disability and death in this country.

There are no guarantees regarding health in this life, and a person can make all the right choices and still encounter a serious injury or illness. However, the evidence is strong that those who do make the wise and correct choices in matters over which they have control will stack the odds in their favor for good health and longevity. So even though making the right health maintenance choices may not be easy, the stakes are so high that the effort is worth it. Physicians need to increase their skills as educators to make this more achievable for their patients. The word *doctor* derives from the Latin *docere,* which means *to teach.*

Another personal effort that can ensure appropriate care is for a patient to assume a more active self-care role in the treatment of certain minor acute problems or chronic conditions that may arise. This was discussed in some depth earlier in this chapter as a partial solution to the physician shortage. There is every reason to believe that this can be done safely and effectively with the information and tools now widely available.

The final area in which individuals can personally increase the likelihood of receiving appropriate medical care involves taking control of their own end-of-life decisions. This benefit is available to virtually everyone who is willing to plan for this inevitable situation. However, too many people simply avoid thinking about it for a variety of reasons. Even many of those who do have a good idea of their preferences do not present these to either their loved ones or their healthcare providers. There are ways to avoid this.

The first is to face this issue as early in life as possible and make the necessary personal decisions required. The second is to have a frank and detailed discussion with family members regarding these decisions. This may be uncomfortable, and it could seem unfair to "burden" your loved ones with this, but it is worse to create a much greater burden if they are faced with the situation of not knowing your wishes when the time comes. A similar discussion needs to occur with any and all current and future healthcare providers.

Finally, these wishes should be legally addressed with specific documents known as advanced directives. This includes a living will and a medical power of attorney. Copies of these documents should be given to appropriate family and healthcare providers.

The final consumer skill required in order to receive appropriate medical care involves making wise, informed, shared decisions when confronted with recommendations from healthcare professionals. The first step in achieving this skill is establishing relationships with only trustworthy healthcare providers as described in the first 10 chapters. In a perfect world this would entail having a primary care provider that would be the source of the majority of care needed, but also provide referrals to ethical specialists if required. In this perfect scenario, every provider involved would be totally up to date, make accurate diagnoses, communicate with all other providers on the case, and clearly lay out all options for treatment with pros and cons for each.

The reality is that this idealized scenario requires a level of perfection that is not realistic—even with the most trustworthy and dedicated healthcare providers. This reality requires following the advice of an old Russian proverb,

JUDSON HENDERSON, M.D
PATRICIA HENDERSON, FNP-BC

"Trust, but verify." This may not be necessary with minor acute medical conditions or even some uncomplicated, stable chronic health problems. However, when there are major problems, it is the only responsible action. The most common option is to request a second or third opinion, as discussed earlier in this book. It is worth repeating here that any trustworthy provider will not be offended when another opinion is requested. It is also true that this verification process is difficult, or sometimes impossible, in the case of an emergency.

A word of caution is appropriate here regarding the use of the internet when seeking medical advice or an "electronic second opinion." This has become known as using "Dr. Google." While there are reliable websites that can provide accurate and valuable information (refer to the references for these in chapter 3), there are far more sites that can misinform and have dangerous results if taken seriously.

This book opened with the question, "Can you trust your doctor?", and we pointed out that the answer is "yes" for the majority of U.S. citizens. Our primary goal has been to reduce the number of persons in the minority for whom the answer is "no." Our healthcare system is facing a crisis on many fronts. A crisis implies deep problems and the actions taken in response can result in chaos and great harm. However, a crisis also presents opportunities for positive change. If this crisis is to produce the latter, it will require engaged and informed healthcare consumers working in partnership with trustworthy and ethical providers that can learn from the past and forge a better system for the future. It is our hope that this book can play a small part in this process.

BIBLIOGRAPHY

Almeida, C M., M A. Rodriguez, S Skootsky, and J Pregler. "Cervical Cancer Screening Overuse and Underuse: Patient and Physician Factors." *American Journal of Managed Care* 19, no. 6 (June 2013): 482-9. https://www.ncbi.nlm.nih.gov/pubmed/23844709.

"AMA Code of Medical Ethics Opinions on Patient-Physician Relationships." JAMA. https://www.ama-assn.org/sites/ama-assn.org/files/corp/media-browser/code-of-medical-ethics-chapter-1.pdf.

Amadeo, Kimberly. "The Rising Cost of Health Care by Year and Its Causes." The Balance. Last modified January 14, 2020. https://www.thebalance.com/causes-of-rising-health care-costs-4064878.

"America's Health Literacy: Why We Need Accessible Health Information." U.S. Department of Health and Human Services. Last modified 2008. https://health.gov/communication/literacy/issuebrief/.

Andrist, Eric. "Dr. Zev-David Nash." The Patient Safety League. Last modified November 2015. http://4patientsafety.org/2015/11/03/dr-zev-david-nash/.

"An Epidemic of Unnecessary Surgeries." Health Link Medical Center. https://healthlinkcenter.com/epidemic-of-unnecessary-surgeries/.

"Antibiotic Prescription Fill Rates Declining in the U.S." Blue Cross Blue Shield. Last modified August 24, 2017. https://www.bcbs.com/the-health-of-america/reports/antibiotic-prescription-rates-declining-in-the-US.

"Antibiotic Use in Outpatient Settings, 2017." Centers for Disease Control and Prevention. Last modified August 8, 2019. https://www.cdc.gov/antibiotic-use/stewardship-report/outpatient.html.

Arthur, Gale. "The Onerous Rules of the American Board of Internal Medicine and the National Quality Forum Reward Bureaucrats, Undermine Physician Morale, and Do Not Improve Patient Care." *Mo Med* 115, no. 4 (July 2018): 316-18. https://www.ncbi.nlm.nih.gov/pmc/articles/PMC6140246/.

Bal, Sonny G. "An Introduction to Medical Malpractice in the United States." *Clinical Orthopaedics and Related Research* 467, no. 2 (November 26, 2008): 339-47. https://doi.org/10.1007/s11999-008-0636-2.

Banks, Gabrielle. "Houston Doctor Sentenced to Prison for Medicare Fraud." *Houston Chronicle*, March 24, 2016. https://www.houstonchronicle.com/news/houston-texas/houston/article/Houston-doctor-sentenced-to-prison-for-Medicare-7045012.php.

Berge, Keith H., Marvin D. Seppala, and Agnes M. Schipper. "Chemical Dependency and the Physician." *Mayo Clinic Proceedings* 84, no. 7 (July 2009): 625-31. https://doi.org/10.1016/S0025-6196(11)60751-9.

Berlin, Joey. "Battling Burnout." Texas Medical Association. Last modified April 2018. https://www.texmed.org/BattlingBurnout/.

Berlin, Joey. "Coming of Age: Celebrating 15 Years of Texas Tort Reform." Texas Medicine. Last modified September 14, 2018. https://doi.org/10.1007/s11999-008-0636-2.

Bullock, Mark. "Doctor Confesses to Faking Flu Shots." WSFA. Last modified July 27, 2005. https://www.wsfa.com/story/4236706/doctor-confesses-to-faking-flu-shots/.

"By the Way, Doctor: Should I Be Tested at Life Line Screening?" Harvard Health. https://www.health.harvard.edu/newsletter_article/By_the_way_doctor_Should_I_be_tested_at_Life_Line_Screening.

Carlson, S A., E K. Adams, Z Yang, and J E. Fulton. "Percentage of Deaths Associated With Inadequate Physical Activity in the United States." *Preventing Chronic Disease* 15 (March 29, 2018). https://doi.org/doi.org/10.5888/pcd18.170354.

"Cervical Cancer Screening FAQ085." The American College of Obstetricians and Gynecologists. Last modified September 2017. https://www.acog.org/Patients/FAQs/Cervical-Cancer-Screening?IsMobileSet=false.

Charlesworth, Christina J., Ellen Smit, David S. Lee, Fatimah Alramadhan, and Michelle C. Odden. "Polypharmacy Among Adults Aged 65 Years and Older in the United States: 1988–2010." *J Gerontol A Biol Sci Med Sci*. 70, no. 8 (August 2015): 989-95. https://doi.org/10.1093/gerona/glv013.

"Christopher Duntsch." Wikipedia. Last modified January 2020. https://en.wikipedia.org/wiki/Christopher_Duntsch.

Consumerism. (2020). In: *Dictionary.com*. [online] Available at: https://www.dictionary.com/browse/consumerism?s=t [Accessed 6 Feb. 2020].

Cook, David A., Morris J. Blachman, Colin P. West, and Christopher M. Wittich. "Physician Attitudes About Maintenance of Certification." *Mayo Clinic Proceedings* 91, no. 10 (October 2016): 1336-45. https://doi.org/10.1016/j.mayocp.2016.07.004.

"Criminal and Civil Enforcement." U.S. Department of Health and Human Services. https://oig.hhs.gov/fraud/enforcement/criminal/.

"Defining the PCMH Home Resource Center." Agency for Healthcare Research and Quality. https://pcmh.ahrq.gov/page/defining-pcmh.

Derbyshire, Robert C. "The Make-Believe Doctors (1993)." Credential Watch. Last modified February 25, 2005. https://www.credentialwatch.org/inv/impostors.shtml.

Doherty, Tucker. "Medicare's Time Bomb, in 7 Charts." *Politico*, September 12, 2018. https://www.politico.com/agenda/story/2018/09/12/medicare-baby-boomers-trust-fund-000694.

"Dr. Joseph Michael Swango." Murderpedia. https://murderpedia.org/male.S/s/swango-michael.htm.

"Economic Cost of Substance Abuse in the United States." Recovery Centers of America. https://recoverycentersofamerica.com/economic-cost-substance-abuse/.

Eisler, Peter. "Doctors, Medical Staff on Drugs Put Patients at Risk." *USA Today*, April 15, 2014. https://www.usatoday.com/story/news/nation/2014/04/15/doctors-addicted-drugs-healthcare-diversion/7588401/.

Evans, Robert G. "Waste, Economists and American Healthcare." *Healthcare Policy* 9, no.

2 (November 2013): 12-20. https://www.ncbi.
nlm.nih.gov/pmc/articles/PMC3999538/.

Gladstone, Jennifer. "Medical Background Checks Lacking."
Ebi. Last modified September 28, 2016. https://www.ebiinc.
com/resources/blog/medical-background-checks-lacking.

"Higher Use of Advanced Imaging Services by
Providers Who Self-Refer Costing Medicare
Millions." United States Government Accountability
Office. Last modified September, 2012. https://
www.gao.gov/assets/650/648988.pdf.

Lowes, Robert. "Medical Board Faulted for Licensing
Convicted Rapist." Medscape. Last modified November 25,
2014. https://www.medscape.com/viewarticle/835430.

Slack, Donovan. "USA TODAY Investigation: VA Knowingly
Hires Doctors with Past Malpractice Claims, Discipline for
Poor Care." *USA Today*, December 3, 2017. https://www.
usatoday.com/story/news/politics/2017/12/03/usa-to-
day-investigation-va-knowingly-hires-doctors-past-mal-
practice-claims-discipline-poor-care/909170001/.

Steinhauer, Jennifer. "Patient Settles Case Of Initials
Cut in Skin." *New York Times*, February 12, 2000.
https://www.nytimes.com/2000/02/12/nyregion/
patient-settles-case-of-initials-cut-in-skin.html.

"Health Literacy Universal Precautions Toolkit, 2nd; Use
the Teach-Back Method: Tool #5 Edition." U.S. Department
of Health and Human Services. Last modified February
2015. https://www.ahrq.gov/health-literacy/quality-re-
sources/tools/literacy-toolkit/healthlittoolkit2-tool5.html.

"Health Savings Accounts and Other Tax-Favored
Health Plans." Department of the Treasury. Last modified 2018. https://www.irs.gov/pub/irs-pdf/p969.pdf.

Japsen, Bruce. "U.S. Doctor Shortage Could Hit 90,000 By 2025." *Forbes*, March 3, 2015. https://www.forbes.com/sites/brucejapsen/2015/03/03/u-s-doctor-shortage-could-hit-90000-by-2025/#3919ae2b9285.

Kale, Minal S., Tara F. Bishop, and Alex D. Federman. ""Top 5" Lists Top $5 Billion." *JAMA Internal Medicine* 171, no. 20 (November 2011): 1858-59. https://doi.org/doi:10.1001/archinternmed.2011.501.

Kamal, Rabah, Daniel McDermott, and Cynthia Cox. "How has U.S. Spending on Healthcare Changed Over Time?" Health System Tracker. Last modified December 20, 2019. https://www.healthsystemtracker.org/chart-collection/u-s-spending-health care-changed-time/#item-nhe-trends_per-capita-out-of-pocket-expenditures-1970-2018.

Kaplan, Deborah A. "Physicians' Battle to Limit Maintenance of Certification Requirements Continues Despite Testing Changes." Medical Economics. Last modified October 2018. https://www.medicaleconomics.com/business/physicians-battle-limit-maintenance-certification-requirements-continues-despite-testing-changes.

Kowarski, Ilana. "How High of a College GPA Is Needed for Med School?" US News. https://www.usnews.com/education/best-graduate-schools/top-medical-schools/articles/2018-10-02/how-high-of-a-college-gpa-is-necessary-to-get-into-medical-school.

"Local Physicians Sentenced Again – Must Pay More Than $37 Million In Restitution." Department of Justice. Last modified April 30, 2015. https://www.justice.gov/usao-sdtx/pr/local-physicians-sentenced-again-must-pay-more-37-million-restitution.

Lyons, Richard D. "2 Medical Schools Closed in Scandal." *The New York Times*, May 16, 1984. https://www.nytimes.com/1984/05/16/us/2-medical-schools-closed-in-scandal.html.

Marrero, Tony. "Victims Disfigured by Unlicensed Town 'N Country Liposuction Center, Authorities Say." *Tampa Bay Times*, April 1, 2017. https://www.tampabay.com/news/publicsafety/crime/two-charged-with-performing-liposuction-without-license-in-town-n-country/2332261/.

"Medicare Fraud Strike Force." U.S. Department of Health and Human Services. https://oig.hhs.gov/fraud/strike-force/.

"National Health Expenditure Data." Centers for Medicare and Medicaid Services. Last modified December 17, 2019. https://www.cms.gov/Research-Statistics-Data-and-Systems/Statistics-Trends-and-Reports/NationalHealthExpendData/NationalHealthAccountsHistorical.

"Obesity: Facts, Figures, Guidelines." West Virginia Department of Health and Human Resources. Last modified December 2002. https://www.wvdhhr.org/bph/oehp/obesity/mortality.htm.

Olinger, David. "Drug-addicted, Dangerous and Licensed for the Operating Room." *Denver Post*, June 2016. https://www.denverpost.com/2016/04/23/drug-addicted-dangerous-and-licensed-for-the-operating-room/.

Ozawa, Sachiko, Allison Portnoy, Hiwote Getaneh, Samantha Clark, and Maria Knoll. "Modeling The Economic Burden Of Adult Vaccine-Preventable Diseases In The United States." *Health Affairs* 35, no. 11. https://doi.org/doi.org/10.1377/hlthaff.2016.0462.

Peters, Philip G. "Twenty Years of Evidence on the Outcomes of Malpractice Claims." *Clinical Orthopaedics and Related Research* 467, no. 2 (February 2009): 352-57. https://doi.org/10.1007/s11999-008-0631-7.

Phillips, Kari A., and Naykky S. Ospina. "Physicians Interrupting Patients." *Journal of the American Medical Association* 318, no. 1 (July 2017): 93-94. https://doi.org/doi:10.1001/jama.2017.6493.

"Radiology Technician Sentenced to 30 Years for Product Tampering." The Federal Bureau of Investigation. Last modified September 11, 2012. https://archives.fbi.gov/archives/jacksonville/press-releases/2012/radiology-technician-sentenced-to-30-years-for-product-tampering.

Rao, T S., and C Andrade. "The MMR vaccine and autism: Sensation, refutation, retraction, and fraud." *Indian Journal of Psychiatry* 53, no. 2 (April 2011): 95-96. https://doi.org/10.4103/0019-5545.82529.

"Reported Cases and Deaths from Vaccine Preventable Diseases, United States, 1950-2005." Centers for Disease Control and Prevention. Last modified May 2019. https://www.cdc.gov/vaccines/pubs/pinkbook/downloads/appendices/E/reported-cases.pdf.

Safaeian, Mahboobeh, Diane Solomon, and Philip E. Castle. "Cervical Cancer Prevention - Cervical Screening: Science in Evolution." *Obstetrics and Gynecology Clinics of North America* 34, no. 4 (December 2007): 739-60. https://doi.org/10.1016/j.ogc.2007.09.004.

Schalit, Naomi. "How Was a Drug-addicted Doctor with Hep C Able to Infect his Patients?" Health and Medicine. *The Conversation*, February 26, 2013. http://theconversation.com/how-was-a-drug-addicted-doctor-with-hep-c-able-to-infect-his-patients-12166.

Schleiter, Kristin E. "Difficult Patient-Physician Relationships and the Risk of Medical Malpractice Litigation." *AMA Journal of Ethics.* https://doi.org/10.1001/virtualmentor.2009.11.3.hlaw1-0903.

"Science Summary: CDC Studies on Thimerosal in Vaccines." Centers for Disease Control and Prevention. https://www.cdc.gov/vaccinesafety/pdf/cdcstudiesonvaccinesandautism.pdf.

Smith, Alexander, Ellen McCarthy, Ellen Weber, Irena S. Cenzer, and John Boscardin. "Half Of Older Americans Seen In Emergency Department In Last Month Of Life; Most Admitted To Hospital, And Many Die There." *Health Aff (Millwood)* 31, no. 6 (June 2012): 1277-85. https://doi.org/10.1377/hlthaff.2011.0922.

Sullivan, Thomas. "Anti-MOC Laws Picking Up Steam Across the United States." Policy Med. Last modified May 4, 2018. https://www.policymed.com/2017/06/anti-moc-laws-picking-up-steam-across-the-united-states.html.

Tavernise, Sabrina. "Antibiotic-Resistant Infections Lead to 23,000 Deaths a Year, C.D.C. Finds." *The New York Times,* September 16, 2013. https://www.nytimes.com/2013/09/17/health/cdc-report-finds-23000-deaths-a-year-from-antibiotic-resistant-infections.html.

"Texans' Experiences with Affordability of and Access to Health Care." Episcopal Health Foundation. Last modified June 2019. https://www.episcopalhealth.org/files/3815/6044/2653/Texans_Experiences_with_Health_Care_Affordability_and_Access_2019_FINALjune.pdf.

"Tobacco-Related Mortality." Centers for Disease Control and Prevention. Last modified 2014. https://

www.cdc.gov/tobacco/data_statistics/fact_sheets/
health_effects/tobacco_related_mortality/index.htm.

The Cost of Dying: End-of-Life Care. Directed by Andy Court, CBS, 2010. DVD.

"The Role of GME Funding in Addressing the Physician Shortage." Association of American Medical Colleges. https://www.aamc.org/news-insights/gme.

"The Scope of Physician Addiction." Physician Health Program. https://www.physicianhealth-program.com/scope-physician-addiction/.

Whitney, Cynthia G., Fangjun Zhou, James Singleton, and Anne Schuchat. "Benefits from Immunization During the Vaccines for Children Program Era — United States, 1994–2013." *Morbidity and Mortality Weekly Report* 63, no. 16 (April 25, 2014): 352-55. https://www.ncbi.nlm.nih.gov/pmc/articles/PMC4584777/.

"Whooping Cough (Pertussis)." National Foundation for Infectious Diseases. https://www.nfid.org/infectious-diseases/pertussis-whooping-cough/.

Worthington, Danika. "Fake Denver Doctor Who Posed as a Plastic Surgeon Sentenced to 6 Years in Prison." *Denver Post*, June 2, 2017. https://www.denverpost.com/2017/06/02/denver-fake-plastic-surgeon-sentenced/.

"2018 Generic Drug Access and Savings Report." Association for Accessible Medicines. https://accessible-meds.org/2018-generic-drug-access-and-savings-report.

"18 Million Avoidable Hospital Emergency Department Visits Add $32 Billion in Costs to the Health Care System Each Year." United Heath Group. Last modified 2019. https://www.unitedhealthgroup.com/content/dam/UHG/PDF/2019/UHG-Avoidable-ED-Visits.pdf.

www.ingramcontent.com/pod-product-compliance
Lightning Source LLC
LaVergne TN
LVHW041640060526
838200LV00040B/1644